D1365324

–the–
eating wisely for
hormonal balance
JOURNAL

A DAILY GUIDE TO HELP YOU
MANAGE YOUR WEIGHT, GAIN ENERGY,
AND ACHIEVE GOOD HEALTH

SONIA GAEMI, ED.D., RD
& MELISSA KIRK

New Harbinger Publications, Inc.

Publisher's Note

This publication is designed to provide accurate and authoritative information in regard to the subject matter covered. It is sold with the understanding that the publisher is not engaged in rendering psychological, financial, legal, or other professional services. If expert assistance or counseling is needed, the services of a competent professional should be sought.

Distributed in Canada by Raincoast Books

Copyright © 2005 by Sonia Gaemi and Melissa Kirk
New Harbinger Publications, Inc.
5674 Shattuck Avenue
Oakland, CA 94609

Cover design by Amy Shoup
Cover image: Getty Images/Stockbyte Platinum
Text design by Michele Waters-Kermes and Amy Shoup
Acquired by Melissa Kirk
Edited by Kayla Sussell

ISBN 1-57224-394-5 Paperback
All Rights Reserved

Printed in the United States of America

New Harbinger Publications' Web site address: www.newharbinger.com

Library of Congress Cataloging-in-Publication Data
Gaemi, Sonia.
    The eating wisely for hormonal balance journal : a daily guide to help you manage your weight, gain energy, and achieve good health / Sonia Gaemi and Melissa Kirk.
        p. cm.
    Includes bibliographical references.
    ISBN 1-57224-394-5
    1. Women—Nutrition—Popular works. 2. Women—Health and hygiene—Popular works. 3. Hormones—Popular works. 4. Diaries. I. Kirk, Melissa. II. Title.
    RA778.G252 2005
    613'.04244—dc22
                                    2005010589

07 06 05

10 9 8 7 6 5 4 3 2 1

First printing

table of contents

table of recipes

acknowledgments

When you dance the whole universe will dance.
—Rumi

I am grateful for Mother Nature's energy, freely given to us by the sun, oxygen, water, and healing tea from the Earth. All are essential for the health of our being.

This small book you hold in your hands is intended as a creative companion to my book *Eating Wisely for Hormonal Balance* and to my qi gong Chinese energy healing exercise DVDs.

I am thankful to thousands of women around the globe who shared their wisdom to give birth to this health and healing model. I am grateful to the Internet and to you for giving me an opportunity to hear from you via my Web site, www.drsonia.com, and for sharing our common wisdom.

I am very grateful to my long-term teachers Master Hui Liu and grandmaster Yang Moijun, as well as my friends and family. I feel deep gratitude to my publishing team, editors, and cowriter Melissa Kirk. Their shared vision for the possibilities of this book as a means of creating harmony for the individual and extending peacefulness to the larger world was especially helpful.

Children are the seeds of our lives. For that reason, I am dedicating this book to my grandchildren: Sophia, Koosha, Leila, Kian, Sasha, and Denna in the hope that they will follow my healing mission, especially to help the children who have suffered so much in the earthquake of Bam/Iran, the 2005 tsunami, and other natural disasters.

I also dedicate this book to the Women for Cultural Wisdom, to my Russian grandmother Habah, the queen of wisdom healing with tea, and to my American mother, Mary Rudge, an international poet laureate and a queen of words in bringing peace to the world. These women believe that healing the world is also self-healing. We must always remember that the Earth is our mother.

In December of 2004, I lost my great teacher, Dr. Sheldon Margen, who cofounded the UC Berkeley Wellness Letter. I dedicate this book to him and to the great master of education, Paolo Freire, who taught that to teach people to teach themselves is the only way to self and world healing.

introduction

Welcome to *The Eating Wisely for Hormonal Balance Journal*. This is the companion journal to the earlier book, *Eating Wisely for Hormonal Balance* (Gaemi 2004), which first introduced the concept of eating hormonally. This journal was designed to help you become your own lifestyle coach by putting the ideas behind eating hormonally into practice in your own life, and by seeing the connection between how you eat, how you approach the world, and your physical and mental health.

Eating hormonally means eating a variety of organic, colorful, whole foods, as well as bringing all of the senses to each meal, focusing on color, aroma, texture, and flavor. Eating hormonally boosts and supports the immune system, which is vital to the healing and prevention of diseases and conditions such as allergies, weight gain, fatigue, colitis, skin conditions, PMS, menopausal symptoms, and diabetes, as well as chronic autoimmune conditions such as lupus, AIDS, multiple sclerosis, and arthritis.

Eating hormonally is about living in balance within our bodies and minds and with the world. The foods you'll be encouraged to eat will be organic, fresh, whole, plant-based foods, organic yogurt and eggs, wild-caught fish, and certain types of soft cheese.

You will be asked to start paying attention to the amazing array of colors that natural foods offer, and to try to eat as many of these colors as you can every day. The movement and "quiet mind" practices will help you see yourself as a part of nature, and will help you balance your energies with the energy of nature and the foods you eat. You'll find that these practices will help you stay calm and centered even during the busiest times of your life. We want you to see that living in balance with nature, including your own nature, as well as taking charge of your own healing, will not only help you and your loved ones to heal, it will help to heal the whole world.

We'll also encourage you to learn more about how different foods affect your hormones, which, in turn, affect your energy levels, moods, and overall health. You'll learn how to be your own personal lifestyle and health coach, using your specific physical condition and mental attitude to make food and lifestyle decisions that are right for you. There is no one "right" food plan; we all have different needs, and this journal will help you discover yours.

With the information you'll learn about yourself in this journal, you'll begin to make changes that will enhance your body's natural hormonal balance and help you to stay healthy and vibrant. As you become more balanced, you'll have more energy and feel more joy, and your creative juices will flow freely as you experiment with all the wonderful, colorful, delicious foods that Mother Nature provides.

In chapter 4 you will see six weeks of journal pages in which you will record your meals, moods, energy levels, goals, and other lifestyle factors. Keeping this journal is your first step in beginning a conversation with your body. You'll discover that your body will tell you what it needs. By listening to it when it aches, is tired or lethargic, or develops symptoms like constipation, bloating, or PMS, you can use this journal to adjust your meals and lifestyle so that you give your body the physical, nutritional, and emotional support it needs to feel healthy, strong, and able to meet your daily challenges. Note that if you have a lot to say in your journal or you have very large handwriting, you may want to keep a separate notebook in addition to the journal pages provided in chapter 4. ❧

is this book for you?

Although we concentrate on women's hormonal, nutritional, behavioral, and physical needs in this journal, it's a myth that men don't also need hormonal balance. Men have hormones, too, and when they eat for balanced hormones they get the same benefits that women do. For that reason, men are also encouraged to use this book. Another myth holds that young people need not be concerned about their hormones. But hormones are active throughout our lives, and they can be out of balance at any time. Many health problems, including depression and other mental illnesses, which can occur at any age, are caused or exacerbated by hormone imbalances.

Eating for hormonal health should begin in the womb, but since we can't control what our mothers ate when we were in the womb, we can begin at any age. For those of us who haven't always taken care to eat wisely and nurture our bodies with a diverse and healthful eating style, it's never too late; and for parents, it's never too early to help your children and other family members acquire wise, joyful eating habits. This book can be especially valuable for women who are pregnant or nursing or are considering becoming pregnant, as well as parents of both sexes. A strong nutritional foundation based on natural whole foods will put any child on a lifelong path of good health. This book will also be useful to all health professionals who need to understand the connections between the foods we eat and the health of our bodies and minds. ❧

eating hormonally for health

Sonia Gaemi developed this program based on her own research and observations of the wisdom of thousands of women all over the world. She found that women in all cultures use the natural healing elements of food to keep themselves, their families, and their communities healthy. In the industrialized societies of the West, we typically eat high-fat, high-calorie foods and live low-activity lifestyles. Until recently, "energy healing" practices like acupressure, qi gong, yoga, tai chi, and other forms of movement meditation that work with the energy flow of the body were dismissed as "too far-out." Lately, however, Western researchers have discovered the healing powers of these practices. The healing properties of herbs and tea also have been endorsed by a once-doubting medical establishment. Western society is slowly coming to realize what the wisdom of women all over the world has told us for generations: the foods we eat and the ways we think and move our bodies can heal or harm us. ❧

foods for life

Did you know that eating foods high in calcium, magnesium, and vitamin D, such as hummus, garbanzo beans, figs, flax seeds, soy nuts, leafy greens like arugula, watercress, spinach, and kale, yogurt, feta cheese, black beans, almonds, and spices such as cumin and fennel seeds can help prevent osteoporosis (Heaney 1993)? Or that studies show that garbanzo beans can prevent or diminish the negative symptoms of menopause, such as hot flashes (Albertazzi et al. 1998), as well as symptoms associated with perimenopause and PMS? Garbanzos have also been shown to lower cholesterol up to 33 percent in humans (Siddiqui and Siddiqui 1976). In another study, organic soy had as much of an effect on estrogenic activity in women test subjects as the synthetic estrogen replacement pill Premarin, without Premarin's negative side effects, such as increased risk of some cancers (Spicer, Shoupe, and Pike 1991.)

We offer tips, suggestions, and ideas for ways to use foods differently, as well as introducing you to foods, herbs, spices, flowers, and herbal teas you may not have used before. You are encouraged to experiment with new foods or recipes, and to record them in this journal along with your feelings, moods, and energy levels before and after your meals. You'll notice that we include several recipes in this book, to show you how delicious eating hormonally can be. We've included all the recipes in an index at the beginning of the book so you can find your favorites again easily. Eating hormonally can be colorful, delicious, fun, and have a profound effect on your life that goes beyond physical health.

YOUR FOOD COLLAGE

The key to eating hormonally and the key to enjoying food is to eat a diversity of colors, textures, and tastes—but often, when we're used to shopping at the same places and making the same meals, we get used to the same foods, day in and day out. In chapter 1, we'll explore the specific elements in food that are important to health, but for now, we'd like to invite you to express your creative and artistic side.

This exercise is designed to help you have fun while imagining yourself as a piece of art composed of healthy foods of all types and colors. It is intended to help you think creatively about food, as well as to recognize the staggering diversity of foods that you have at your disposal. Using a separate piece of paper, create a collage of all the types of whole foods you can think of. It might be helpful to go over the Food Wisdom Pyramid in chapter 1 and jot down all the types of food in each category that come to mind.

Your collage can be as large or small as you want it, and you can use any medium: crayons, colored pencils and pens, paints, pictures from magazines and food packaging, or anything that strikes your fancy. Challenge yourself to find new and unfamiliar foods to represent in the collage, such as flaxseeds, bitter melon, fenugreek, pomegranate, or dandelion greens. If you're feeling stuck, visit your local supermarket, natural foods store, farmer's market, or local ethnic market. Make a note of foods you're unfamiliar with, or even sketch them or describe their color and shape for your collage. The point is to become mindful of the infinite variety of colors, textures, tastes, and smells of food. When you're done, hang your piece of art in the kitchen where you will see it every day and it will remind you to approach your meals as you would a painter's canvas, with creativity and imagination.

KEEPING A JOURNAL

Studies have shown that journaling can be healing. Researchers have discovered that journaling strengthens the immune system and can lower blood pressure (Pennebaker 1997). Journaling researchers believe that the act of writing helps the brain to process information more quickly because it allows us to use both sides of our brain—the thinking and the feeling sides—simultaneously. This journal will help you to understand the role of food in your life and health, and help you break out of eating patterns that cause you to have food cravings, lose or gain excess weight, be at risk for certain health problems, have unhealthy skin, a compromised immune system, problems with your metabolism, or low energy.

This is *your* food journal. Use it however you see fit, but remember to remain curious and open-minded. Many "weight-loss" diaries and diet-tracking journals make you feel guilty if you miss a day, eat a favorite sweet for dessert, or comfort yourself with a food not on your diet. This journal is different. There is no guilt here. You are responsible for your own health, and we hope you will discover how the benefits of eating hormonally, including taking pleasure in your food, will improve your life and health. ❧

what you'll find in this book

Chapter 1 introduces the Food Wisdom Pyramid, designed by Sonia Gaemi as an alternative to the U. S. Department of Agriculture food pyramid. Based on Sonia's years of research into how women from all over the world use food to keep themselves, their families, and their communities healthy, this pyramid relies on plant foods, including greens, grains, legumes, herbs, seeds, nuts, fruits, and spices; and animal foods such as yogurt, eggs, fish, and soft cheeses like feta, ricotta, and cottage cheese. We encourage you to use meat and other high-fat foods for flavoring but not as the main part of your meals. The pyramid also includes elements not usually viewed as food, but that serve as the building blocks of all food: sunlight, oxygen, and water.

You can use the pyramid to design your own menu for any meal and be confident that you're feeding and supporting your body and mind. You'll learn to build your own food pyramid based on your likes and dislikes, and you'll be challenged to use unfamiliar foods and to experiment with new recipes and food combinations.

Chapter 2 describes how you can become your own lifestyle and healing coach by deciding on what you want to accomplish with this food journal. Do you want to heal a particularly troubling symptom, feel more energetic, have a healthy baby, or enjoy more beautiful skin and hair? We all have different needs, and chapter 2 will help you decide what your needs are and how to use this journal to help yourself stay energetic and healthy.

Chapter 3 describes using the food journal, the heart of this book. When you track your energy levels, mood and thoughts on waking, the pleasure you get from your meals, your physical exercise, movement meditation or other "quiet mind" practices for the day, the foods you ate, how you felt at the meal and after it, and your personal and meal goals for the next day, you will arrive at a better understanding about how the foods you eat affect your hormones, immune system, metabolism, moods, and how you feel from hour to hour.

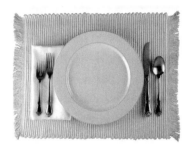

The food journal pages in chapter 4 are the heart of this book. Remember that tracking your food, energy level, breathing, movement, and moods and thoughts during the day should be fun. The insights you will gain will change the way you approach your meals, your body, and your entire way of being. Remember, you are the only one who can give yourself the gifts of vibrant health and well-being. And one way to do this is by eating hormonally.

If you skip a day of writing in your food journal, that's okay. This journal is only a tool. There is no wrong way to approach it, so long as you start from this moment. Even if you don't use the food journal consistently, it will still be useful. Approach it as you would a loved one: with sensitivity and a sense of fun. You'll be recording the story of your mental, physical, and spiritual growth in these pages. Be patient and allow the healing process to emerge.

Chapter 5 deals with making changes in your lifestyle so that, rather than feeling restricted, you can achieve balance and serenity. Changing a lifetime of eating habits, mental habits, and lifestyle habits won't happen overnight. We won't ask you to stop eating all of your favorite foods, but as you learn to eat hormonally, to listen to your body and mind, and to become your own lifestyle coach, you'll learn how to create balance and diversity in your life. In chapter 5, we offer tips and suggestions on how to begin making changes to your lifestyle, how to stick with those changes, and how to enjoy yourself while you explore eating hormonally.

THE KEY IS ENJOYMENT

Enjoyment is the key to any well-lived life. Many people have a love-hate relationship with food. They think that if they enjoy food too much, they will become overweight. They restrict their calorie intake obsessively, or binge on food when they are stressed or unhappy, and then feel guilty afterward. These behaviors can lead to harmful eating disorders, such as anorexia, bulimia, or overeating. We know that dieting does not work in the long run. We may lose weight at first, but once we resume eating the way we ate before the diet, we often gain the weight back. This regained weight is then harder to lose, so people who diet frequently are often more overweight than they would be if they had never dieted.

Eating hormonally is about pleasureful eating, not dieting, calorie counting, restriction, or guilt. When you eat wisely, you feed both your body and mind, approaching every new day with excitement and energy, in the spirit of self-exploration. This way of eating encourages you to be mindful of both your food intake and your lifestyle. It teaches you skills and gives you tools to use for balancing and calming your whole self. When you finish with this journal, be sure to keep it as a reference, as well as a reminder that you have the power to heal yourself.

the food wisdom pyramid, phytohormones, and healing

In the introduction, you were asked to make a food collage where you gathered together all the colors of the rainbow onto the page. That exercise was designed to stimulate your creativity, to show you that eating hormonally can be an act of creating art. Now, we will discuss all the elements in the foods that make them healthful. You will find that eating with a diversity of colors, textures, tastes, and nutrients can be as creative and artistic as your food collage, only this time, your own body and mind are the works of art you are creating. 🪽

the food wisdom pyramid

This chapter introduces you to the Food Wisdom Pyramid and shows you how to use it to develop better health; to stabilize your hormones, metabolism, immune system, mood, and energy levels;

and to prevent or heal adverse health conditions. The Food Wisdom Pyramid developed by Sonia Gaemi is based on research done on foods used all over the world. Unlike the pyramid popularized by the U. S. Department of Agriculture, the Food Wisdom Pyramid includes water, oxygen, and sunlight in addition to food because these elements produce the wonderful bounty that Mother Nature provides. The Food Wisdom Pyramid also focuses on healing tea, phytohormones, essential fats, plant protein, and fiber, and introduces certain seeds as important sources of soluble fiber.

Notice that the pyramid is upside down. This unusual position emphasizes the most critical aspect of the Food Wisdom Pyramid: balance. Balance is the key to good health. This pyramid can be used as a starting point for anyone seeking to eat for better health. Later, you'll design your own personalized pyramid, based on your specific tastes, wellness goals, mood and energy patterns, and health needs

The best way to change any habit is to develop and enjoy your new habit, and this is especially true for eating habits. By

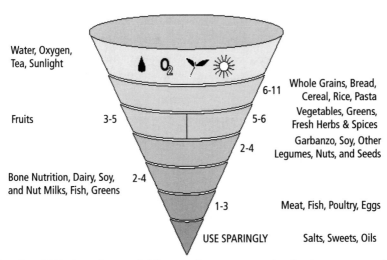

The Food Wisdom Pyramid: The numbers next to the foods represent the number of suggested servings per day, although you don't have to eat them every day if you get the average amount in a week. For example, you can eat 28 servings of fruit in a week and still go one day without eating fruit.

keeping this journal and designing a pyramid that includes a variety of your favorite healthy foods, you will enjoy eating hormonally, and in time you'll enjoy trying new foods and adding them to your pyramid. ❧

the elements of the pyramid

The Food Wisdom Pyramid introduces elements that aren't found in other food pyramids. Here we'll discuss the reasons why these elements are so important to good health and mental and physical vitality.

THE IMPORTANCE OF SUNLIGHT

As you can see on the Food Wisdom Pyramid, the top layer is oxygen, tea, water, and sunlight. Oxygen, water, and sunlight are all required elements for life itself. These are not only necessary in their most basic forms, they also are necessary to grow the foods we eat. Drinking enough water and tea, spending time outdoors to get vitamin D from the sun, and ensuring that your body gets as much oxygen as it can absorb are all important to self-healing.

Clearly, we all need water and oxygen, but not so long ago, the media advised us to avoid the sun at all costs. More recently, studies have emphasized that vitamin D, found in sunlight, is essential to good health, especially for our bones, and that we should enjoy fifteen minutes of sunshine a day to get enough vitamin D (Garland 2003).

The lack of exposure to sunlight has been linked to the childhood bone disease called "rickets" (Hess and Unger 1921), as well as to heart disease (Johnson 1935), some forms of cancer (John et al. 1999), multiple sclerosis (Hayes, Cantorna, and DeLuca 1997), and diabetes (Eurodiab 1999). The sun's rays are also important for another reason: they keep our environment dry. Dampness encourages the growth of mold, viruses, and bacteria. Dryness and warmth often heal or alleviate illnesses brought on by damp.

Sunlight is also good for your mood. All over the world, millions of people experience seasonal affective disorder, or SAD, which usually affects people during the winter months when the sun is hidden by clouds and is lower in the sky. People with SAD feel depressed and lethargic, but when they are exposed to sunlight or to indoor lighting designed to deliver the same type of light as a sunny day, their symptoms disappear.

Enjoy sunlight safely when you can, and be sure to eat foods rich in vitamin D, such as greens, fish, oysters, fortified yogurt, or fortified soy, almond, or rice milk. Also, eat foods high in antioxidants (substances that protect cells from the damaging effects of free radicals, which are thought to play a role in aging, some cancers, and autoimmune disorders). You can also take organic vitamin D supplements, balanced with a supplement of calcium and magnesium, and eat fortified cereals. The best way to get vitamin D, however, is to eat a diverse diet of foods high in fiber, protein, antioxidants, essential fatty acids, and phytohormones, and to take in sunlight whenever you can, taking care to wear an organic sunscreen, a hat, and sunglasses, and not to get sunburned. A good rule of thumb is to avoid the sun between the hours of 11 A.M. to 1 P.M.

THE ANCIENT HEALING ART OF TEA

One of the best ways to get all the benefits of oxygen, water, and sunlight is to drink tea, and eating hormonally uses tea as a vital source of healing. Tea is made from plants rich in antioxidants, phytohormones, vitamins, and minerals absorbed from the earth, air, water, and sun. Tea can be custom-blended for your specific needs by adding berries, flowers, seeds, spices, and herbs. For thousands of years, tea has been used by people all over the world to increase their health and vitality. For example, drinking warming Peaceful & Happy Tea (see recipe below) during cold weather can help cleanse the body and keep your immune system strong and your body warm.

Tea drinkers who consume one to eight cups of black, green, or oolong tea a day lower their risk of stroke, certain cancers, and heart disease (Dufresne and Farnworth 2001). Some tannins found in tea are effective antibiotic agents, and tea also contains fluoride, which helps teeth to remain healthy. The tea recipes provided in this book and online at www.drsonia.com are based on research done on tea, flowers, and herbs and how they affect the body's hormones, moods, metabolism, immune system, and internal organs.

Tea can be used as a healing food by adding herbs, leaves, spices, berries, seeds, and flowers, and it can be used both to heal and prevent health problems. If you feel a cold coming on, just cut up some fresh ginger and a pinch of licorice root and steep them in a cup of hot water. Drinking this ginger tea all day long will help your body fight the cold virus. All types of tea have proved to be excellent sources of phytohormones and antioxidants that can fight infection, help reduce the risk of certain cancers, and improve immune system functioning (Dufresne and Farnworth 2001).

Tea can be used as a meditation aid, or to help you center and calm yourself before and while you write in your journal. Including tea in

Peaceful & Happy Tea

This calming and fortifying tea developed by Sonia Gaemi is a unique infusion of flowers and spices that will please your taste buds. She recommends it for clients suffering from depression, anxiety, low energy, and weight problems. Take the time to breathe in the wonderful steam, letting your lungs expand as you inhale the aroma of the tea. Take a sip and savor the taste and heat in your mouth, and congratulate yourself for taking this moment for healing. The ingredients are as follows:

1 tsp. each of green or jasmine tea, rose petals, rooibos tea, dandelion leaves, lemon balm, chamomile flowers, crushed or sliced ginger, roasted brown rice and/or borage flowers (optional)

½ cup fresh mint or 1 tsp. dried peppermint leaves (optional)

Pinch of orange zest

Mix the ingredients together. Bring 2 cups of water to a boil. Add a large pinch of the tea blend (more to taste) and steep 2–5 minutes. Sweeten with honey and/or natural licorice or ginger candy, if desired, and/or serve with dates.

your life, in addition to eating hormonally and taking time out of your busy day to center your heart and soul, can be a powerful life-changing tool. Instead of coffee, soda, or empty-calorie snacks, make tea your snack and beverage of choice and you'll soon see a difference in how you feel.

Because water is the primary ingredient in tea, know where your water comes from. To find out which water-borne contaminants may be in your water, contact your local water agency and then buy filters specific to the contaminants you want to eliminate. Water filters can attach to your tap or can be freestanding containers with built-in filters. Be sure your water filters bear the seal of NSF International, a nonprofit public health and safety organization.

HERBS AND SPICES

Spices have a history as colorful and diverse as the spices themselves. Early explorers like Columbus and Magellan were looking for new trade routes for spices when they set out on their travels. Spices are excellent sources of healthy nutrients, minerals, and phytohormones, and they are a wonderful way to create beautiful, colorful, aromatic, delicious meals. The Food Wisdom Pyramid is the only food pyramid to include herbs and spices as a necessary food group, and the medicinal properties of herbs and spices are just now beginning to revolutionize how we look at health and nutrition.

Garlic, one of the most popular and widely used plants on the planet, is famed for its ability to boast the immune system. Turmeric and ginger are used worldwide as anti-inflammatory and antibacterial agents, and recent research has shown that turmeric may help to reduce inflammation (Satoskar, Shah, and Shenoy 1986) and cystic fibrosis (Egan et al. 2004). One study has shown that cinnamon has insulin-like properties and can lower blood glucose levels, important for diabetics (Jarvill-Taylor, Anderson, and Graves 2001). Some spices, like cardamom and ginger, can kill up to fifteen different harmful bacterial species (Sherman and Billings 1998). Fenugreek, a leafy green herb, is used worldwide to aid digestion.

In addition to being healthful, herbs and spices taste and smell great, add color to food, and are fun to experiment with. You can include herbs and spices in your food by cutting up fresh parsley, basil, watercress, arugula, and cilantro and adding them to salads or salad dressings. Add fresh mint and rose petals to your tea, a cup of hot water, or yogurt. Chop up fresh green onion and chives for soups, omelets, or bean or rice dishes, and sprinkle fresh oregano, tarragon, sage, and thyme into sauces. Insert a cinnamon stick into a whole apple and microwave for three minutes for a delicious, easy dessert that tastes great with Denna's Rooibos Chai tea (see recipe in chapter 2). You'll find that each spice gives a different character to food, and that combining spices gives you even more options. Try experimenting by using two new herbs or spices a week in your tea, cereals, yogurt, sauces, soups, and salads, and add the ones you love to your personal food pyramid.

In most American households, sugar and salt are probably the most commonly used spices. It's fine to use them, but it's important to know that they can cause health problems if used excessively. There are other, healthier options to season your foods. Organic raw honey, molasses, and licorice root are good sweeteners and lemon and sumac powder can be good substitutes for salt. Avoid artificial sweeteners such as Nutrasweet as much as possible. Use fresh and dried fruit for those sweet cravings, and use

Heart-Healthy Spice Mix

Mix together the following ingredients in a glass container and pour into a salt shaker to use whenever you want to add flavor to your food. To help absorb moisture, add a few grains of uncooked rice to the salt shaker. The ingredients can be found at Middle Eastern or natural food stores.

2 tbsp. dried sumac powder

I tbsp. each of crushed seaweed, green tea leaves, cumin seeds, grape seeds, dried crushed lemon balm leaves, and dried sorrel

Pinch of sea salt

spices and herbs to flavor food instead of salt. The Heart-Healthy Spice Mix is a pungent blend that can be used as you would use salt. ❧

the healing elements of food

This section discusses the most important elements and compounds available in whole foods; how they help us to heal and stay healthy; and which foods we should eat to get more of them. As you track your food intake, movement, energy, moods, and healing goals in your journal, challenge yourself to eat foods that will provide all the elements that are essential to your continued good health. Also, make it a goal to benefit from the healing properties of water, oxygen, sunlight, and tea.

PHYTOHORMONES

Many people believe that only women approaching menopause need to worry about hormonal balance, but this is not true. Regardless of our sex or age, our bodies need hormonal balance. Hormones regulate weight, moods, lifelong health, physical growth, and puberty, so it's important for us to eat wisely for hormonal balance throughout our lives.

Phytohormones are hormonelike compounds found in plants (*phyto* means "plant" in Greek). These elements have weak estrogen-like effects on the body, and may benefit women experiencing estrogen fluctuations due to the onset of puberty, menopausal changes, PMS, pregnancy, or other health changes, without the harmful effects of synthetic estrogen replacements. Phytohormones are particularly important for women before and during pregnancy and as they age, because women's bodies process and eliminate hormones differently during these times and it's easy for our hormones to become unbalanced.

Some foods high in phytohormones include berries, red clover leaves and flowers, dandelion, cumin, turmeric, pomegranate, rooibos tea, garbanzo beans, hummus, tofu, licorice root, thyme, sage, soy, rose petals and hips, wild yams, flax and sesame seeds, and the medicinal herb, black cohosh and dong quai.

NUTRIENT-DENSE FOODS

The Food Wisdom Pyramid focuses on plant-derived foods that provide a good balance of protein, fiber, essential fats, and phytohormones, such as grains, greens, colorful fruits and vegetables, spices, nuts and seeds, legumes, and herbs, as well as animal-based foods, such as yogurt, fish, eggs, and cheeses like feta, mozzarella, and ricotta. These foods are nutrient-dense, meaning that they are high in nutrients. Simple carbohydrates and sugars, such as those found in potato chips and pastries, are calorie-dense, but they are "empty" calories; that is, they are high in calories but low in nutrients.

Although the pyramid focuses mostly on plant foods, meats and hard cheeses (like cheddar and Swiss cheese) are fine to add to a meal when used to flavor to the meal rather than as the main dish. The Food Wisdom Pyramid also emphasizes foods known to have healing or preventive properties for body and mind. This pyramid includes certain seeds, especially flax, basil, black sesame, and psyllium, as these seeds can be important sources of nutrients. They also can function as cleansing agents to rid our bodies of free radicals and excess cholesterol (see chapter 3).

Why Counting Calories Isn't Helpful

Many diet plans ask you to count the calories of every morsel of food you eat, but we believe that it is better to focus on eating a diversity of whole foods (preferably organic) rather than worry about how many calories you are consuming. Calories are not necessarily a good measure of how healthful a food is. For example, each of these foods contains about 80 calories: one egg; one slice of bread; one ounce of meat or cheese; a half a cup of yogurt; two medium-sized pieces of fruit; and a half a cup of rice or beans.

But many of these foods contain other nutrients essential for good health, while eating several potato chips, a pastry, or cookies also equaling 80 calories will provide only fat, sugar, starch, salt, and oil. In a diet where you count calories, eating the potato chips would count for as many calories as two medium-sized pieces of fruit, even though the fruit provides the fiber, antioxidants, and minerals that your body needs. Many people think using artificial sweeteners in their foods and beverages means they are consuming fewer calories, but these sweeteners can induce your body to crave more of them, and we don't know the effects of these artificial additives on our health. It's best to avoid all artificial sweeteners, as well as hydrogenated fats (also called transfats) and excess salt. If you eat a diverse and balanced diet of natural whole foods, your food will naturally be low in calories and high in nutrients. That's why we don't emphasize calories in the eating hormonally program.

THE GLYCEMIC INDEX

How many times have you eaten a sugary snack, felt energetic for a while, and then suddenly felt fatigued? This is because the glucose and simple carbohydrates in those snacks break down quickly and they don't provide lasting nutrients to your body, causing the level of insulin in your blood to diminish. The glycemic index was introduced by the Glycemic Research Institute in 2002. It rates foods based on how quickly they break down into glucose in the bloodstream (Foster-Powell, Holt, and Brand-Miller 2002).

Foods high on the glycemic index are usually the highest in sugar and starch and tend to break down faster, offering sudden but short-lived bursts of energy. High glycemic index foods are often high-calorie, low-nutrient foods like starches, sweets, and "junk" snack foods. They can be useful when you need quick energy, but they tend to leave your body just as quickly, causing an energy "crash" because they don't provide long-term nutrients.

Medium- and low-glycemic foods, such as beans, apples, pears, and yogurt, usually include more protein, complex carbohydrates, essential fatty acids, and fiber, and they break down more slowly in the body, keeping insulin levels steady and thus providing more long-term energy. Often, they cause us to feel more full, and this sense of fullness lasts longer than the "sugar high" of high-glycemic foods. Feeling full for a longer time prevents food cravings and unhealthy weight gain.

The Food Wisdom Pyramid and the eating hormonally program are based on medium- and low-glycemic foods, which are limited in simple carbohydrates and saturated fats but high in complex carbohydrates, essential fatty acids, and fiber, and provide an overall healthy way of eating. A simplified version of the glycemic index follows, but you can find out more online by visiting www.glycemic.com. For most of your meals, make sure you choose foods from the medium and low sections of the glycemic index, and include foods that provide essential fats such as nuts, olives, avocados, seeds, and olive oil. Note that although meat and some other foods high in saturated fats, like hard cheese, are considered low on the glycemic index, they should be used sparingly as side dishes or to add flavoring to a main vegetable-based dish.

High-glycemic foods: Sugar, soda, cornflakes, carrots, potatoes, pretzels, Rice Krispies, jelly beans, parsnips, candy bars, white rice, rice cakes, plain bagel, orange juice, white bread, French fries, saltines, Cheerios, French bread

Medium-glycemic foods: Raisins, beets, semolina pasta, oatmeal muffins, sweet potatoes, corn, yams, brown rice, popcorn (without flavorings), potato chips, whole wheat bread

Low-glycemic foods: Navy beans, dried peas, whole-grain pasta, oranges, baked beans, bran, buckwheat, soba noodles, sprouted or whole garbanzos, pears, apples, milk, yogurt, kidney beans, lentils, barley, soybeans, peanuts, hummus, tofu

Note that carrots and parsnips, although high-glycemic foods, also include fiber, antioxidants, and other important nutrients, so they are recommended. Potato chips, although medium-glycemic foods, are high in fat, salt, and starch, and so are not recommended. Spaghetti can be a healthy food if you eat whole wheat, spinach, or other pasta not made from processed white semolina flour.

ANTIOXIDANTS FOR YOUTH AND IMMUNITY

Free radicals are by-products of the body's normal cellular processes. It is thought they may be carcinogenic and also may contribute to the aging process. *Antioxidants* are substances that deactivate free radicals before they can cause damage. Although study is still ongoing on the effects of antioxidants on various health problems, preliminary findings suggest that they may lower the risk of heart disease, diabetes, some cancers, and stroke, and may help with countering some of the harmful effects of smoking, taking drugs, and drinking. Also, they may help those with impaired autoimmune systems to remain healthy, and they may help counteract the effects of sun damage, pollution, and other harsh elements that cause wrinkles and skin damage. (See the recipe for Sonia's Antioxidant Smoothie later in this chapter, as well as the cleansing plan in chapter 3.) If you take antioxidant supplements like flaxseed oil or fish oil capsules, also make sure to get the more complete forms of antioxidants found in whole foods like those listed below.

Good sources of antioxidants, in the form of vitamins C and E, beta-carotene, selenium, folic acid, and others, include all types of tea (especially green tea and rooibos tea), plums, pomegranates, blueberries, rose hips, hibiscus, blackberries, strawberries, seaweed, green peppers, broccoli, kale, collard greens, Asian pears, raw cabbage, potatoes, whole grains, wheat germ, nuts, seeds, carrots, squash, sweet potatoes, tomatoes, cantaloupe, peaches, fish, shellfish, grains, eggs, turmeric, flaxseeds, sesame seeds, and garlic.

PROTEIN

Every cell in our bodies contains protein, and the health of our muscles, tendons, and ligaments is maintained with protein. Amino acids build protein, but different foods have different amino acids, so it's important to eat a wide variety of foods to get as many types of protein in your diet as possible. Too much protein, however, can negatively affect the kidneys (Wrone et al. 2003) and bones (Feskanich et al. 1996). Try to make protein 10 to 20 percent of your diet (or about 1 gram of protein per kilo or 2.2 pounds of body weight).

As you can see, eating hormonally means getting most of your protein from plants. However, if you like meat, small portions of organic meat can add flavor and protein to your meals. Many cultures use small amounts of lamb, pork, or chicken to flavor dishes of soy, brown rice, buckwheat, black beans, lentils, or garbanzos. Small amounts of animal protein give the meal an appetizing taste without large amounts of saturated fat and cholesterol. Similarly, hard cheeses like cheddar, Swiss, and Parmesan should be used only in small amounts for flavor. Good vegetable sources of protein include sprouts, hummus, tahini, lentils, leafy greens, amaranth, quinoa, peanuts, pumpkin seeds, almonds, seaweed, and tofu. Other sources include yogurt and soft cheese like feta, ricotta, or cottage cheeese.

Eggs, another good source of protein, can be eaten safely several times a week by most people who lead active lives, eat enough fiber, and have good cholesterol levels. Egg whites are a good alternative for those with high cholesterol, although such people should also make sure to cut down on animal foods, eat more fiber and complex carbohydrates, and get more exercise; they may also benefit from yoga, qi gong, or other form of movement meditation. Eggs are a good alternative to soy protein. Eating too much soy can cause health problems. (See the section "The Noble Garbanzo" below.) Eggs can be used in smoothies, eaten hard- or soft-boiled, or scrambled in a pan with a small amount of olive oil and whatever greens, spices, and vegetables you enjoy. Try adding sprouted garbanzos, red clover, or lentils to your egg dish.

Protein and Sleep

If you suffer from insomnia or other sleep interruptions, try adding protein foods to your breakfast and lunch, and then have an early dinner with a focus on fiber and complex carbohydrates like greens, grains, and seaweed, but with little protein. One exception to this is yogurt, which can aid relaxation. Try eating yogurt before bedtime to help with insomnia.

THE NOBLE GARBANZO

The garbanzo bean is an excellent source of phytohormones. In a study that Sonia led at the University of California at Berkeley (Ghaemi-Hashemi, Clarke, and Margen 1998), thirty-three menopausal women not on hormone replacement therapy (HRT) were asked to add one cup of cooked, sprouted, or roasted garbanzos or garbanzo flour to their diets for eight weeks. The subjects reported the rate and intensity of adverse symptoms of menopause were significantly reduced (70 percent reported a reduction in symptoms like hot flashes, anxiety, and constipation by the eighth week). This study indicates that adding garbanzos to your diet can result in positive health benefits. Further studies are ongoing.

Garbanzo beans have been found to lower blood cholesterol, which also affects estrogen, by as much as 35 percent (Siddiqui and Siddiqui 1976). It is thought that the saponins found in garbanzos, soy, and other legumes may lower cholesterol by causing the body to excrete it or by blocking its absorption. However, soy products can cause allergic reactions or food sensitivities in some people, due to incorrect fermentation as well as to the fact that most of the soybean crop in the U.S. has been genetically altered. If you are allergic to soy, then garbanzos are an excellent alternative.

Here's a great way to use garbanzo beans in a tasty dish that you can eat all day long. This is a great bone food that also

Essential Hummus

Make enough to last for several days; the flavor improves with time. If garbanzo beans give you gas, use sprouted garbanzos (see a method for sprouting your own garbanzos at the end of this recipe). This recipe makes 4 to 6 servings.

> **2½ cups cooked or canned, drained garbanzos, or sprouted garbanzos***
>
> **1 cup soft tofu, drained (about 5 ounces) (optional)**
>
> **1 cup yogurt or ricotta cheese**
>
> **½ cup tahini or sesame seeds**
>
> **½ cup ground flaxseeds and/or black sesame seeds**
>
> **¼ cup olive oil**
>
> **¼ cup fresh lemon juice**
>
> **½ cup each of chopped fresh parsley, tarragon, and/or red pepper (optional)**
>
> **½ medium red onion diced (optional)**
>
> **2-3 cloves fresh garlic (optional)**
>
> **1 tsp. cayenne pepper or to taste**
>
> **1 tbsp. tumeric**
>
> **Salt and black pepper to taste**

Combine all ingredients in the bowl of a food processor or blender and puree until smooth. You may need to do this in batches.

Season to taste with lemon juice, salt, and pepper.

Garnish with fresh mint, olives, olive oil, cayenne pepper, paprika, or garbanzo sprouts as desired.

Serve with Healthy & Wise Tea (see recipe in chapter 3)

** **To make sprouted garbanzos,** soak garbanzo beans in water for 2 days, changing the water 2 to 3 times a day. Drain the water and put the beans into a cotton cheesecloth bag, a plastic bag, or a glass jar, and refrigerate. The beans should sprout in 2 days. Use them in pilaf, omelets, salads, hummus, sandwiches, stews, or soups, or eat them raw as snacks. This sprouting method also works with lentils and mung beans. Sprouted garbanzos are useful to balance digestive enzymes and to provide antioxidants.*

provides protein, essential fats, phytohormones, and fiber. It can be used as a dip, a spread, or a salad dressing.

ESSENTIAL FATTY ACIDS: THE GOOD FATS

The human body does not manufacture essential fatty acids (EFAs), such as omega-3 and omega-6, we must get them through our food. A healthy intake of EFAs lowers the risk of certain cancers (Serraino and Thompson 1992), Alzheimer's (Simopoulos 1988), insulin imbalance (Pelikanova et al. 1989), arthritis (Andersen-Parrado 1996), and depression (Logan 2003).

EFAs are one of the foundations of the Food Wisdom Pyramid. Good sources of EFAs include fish, especially wild-caught salmon and light canned tuna, hummus, flaxseeds, eggs, walnuts, almonds and almond butter, sunflower and sesame seeds and their oils, tahini, soy products, avocado, olives, olive paste, olive oil, wheat germ, rice bran, and beans.

It's best to get your EFAs from whole foods rather than supplements. Try using hummus, tahini, olive oil or paste, avocado, or almond butter instead of butter or margarine, and flavor your foods with herbs and spices rather than salt. Harmful hydrogenated fats (also called trans fats) are found in processed foods like margarine, potato chips, cookies, and junk food. Try to limit your intake of fatty meats as well as diet foods with "fake" fats like olestra.

A Word about Fish

Recently, there have been reports that all types of fish are contaminated with mercury to some degree (Environmental Protection Agency 2004). Although this is troubling, it is still possible to eat fish without endangering yourself and, in fact, fish still provides one of the best ways to get EFAs and other nutrients. According to the Federal Food and Drug Administration, salmon and canned light tuna are generally low in mercury, although albacore tuna and tuna steaks have higher levels. Eat wild-caught

Baked Salmon on a bed of Dandelion

This recipe makes enough for 4-6 people. Increase or decrease the recipe according to how many people are eating.

Fish Sauce

> **3 cloves garlic, crushed or minced**
>
> **2-3 tbsp. olive oil**
>
> **½ cup dry white wine (optional)**
>
> **½ cup fresh lemon juice**
>
> **1-2 tsp. crushed chile pepper**
>
> **2 tbsp. capers**
>
> **Pinch of turmeric or saffron (optional)**
>
> **1 tsp. sea salt**
>
> **1 bunch (4 cups) fresh, washed dandelion leaves**
>
> **1 lb. salmon fillet**

Preheat the oven to 375°F. Mix all the sauce ingredients together. Line a baking pan with dandelion leaves. Place the salmon fillets on top of the dandelion leaves. Drizzle the fish sauce on top. Bake for 25 to 30 minutes, or until the fish is tender and flaky, brushing frequently with more sauce. Place a bed of dandelion leaves on each plate and top with a portion of the salmon fillet. Drizzle the pan juices over the fish and serve with steamed buckwheat or Green Garbanzo Dill Pilaf (see chapter 5).

salmon or canned chunk light tuna packed in water two to three times a week. That will ensure you get enough omega-3 fatty acids in your diet. The FDA recommend avoiding shark, swordfish, king mackerel, and tilefish due to high mercury levels. For more information about seafood mercury levels, visit the FDA Web site at www.fda.gov; also see chapter 3 for a cleansing plan to rid your system of accumulated toxins.

COMPLEX CARBOHYDRATES AND FIBER

Recently, carbohydrates have been labeled a "bad food." Low- and no-carb diets are touted as the latest "health miracle." But carbohydrates are not the enemy. Rather, they are an important element your body needs to be healthy, strong, and energetic. Simple carbohydrates are composed of sugar and starch without fiber, and when we're told never to eat bread, tortillas, or chips, these simple carbs are the target.

It's true that too many simple carbohydrates can lead to weight gain. However, complex carbohydrates, which are usually packed with fiber, are important for good health. Complex carbs include whole-grain breads, whole-grain pastas, peas, sprouts, garbanzos, dried berries, soy products, and brown rice. A deficiency in complex carbohydrates (in the form of fiber) has been linked to heart disease (Pereira et al. 2004), diabetes (Liu et al. 2000), and diverticulitis (Idoori et al. 1998). Some foods that are advertised as low-carb, such as low-carb bagels, may include added elements such as fats or protein to make them palatable.

Fiber

Fiber is found in plant foods, and although only a small amount of it is digested, its presence in the body provides extensive health benefits. Fiber is another important element of eating hormonally. There are two types. Both types of fiber are essential for the Eating Hormonally Cleansing Plan, outlined in chapter 3. *Soluble fiber* is found in fruit pectin, oats, dried beans, barley, apples, carrots, garbanzos, most soy products, lentils, some spices and herbs, psyllium, flaxseeds, basil seeds, and some flowers. This type of fiber binds with fatty acids to help reduce the buildup of "bad" cholesterol and other accumulated toxins and helps to regulate insulin levels.

Insoluble fiber, such as that found in leafy greens, whole wheat products, corn bran, green beans, cauliflower, seeds and seed husks, and the skins of fruits and vegetables does not break down in the body at all, and its bulk helps move waste through the intestine. Most whole fruits, vegetables, and grains have both types of fiber, and if you're eating a diverse array of whole foods, you needn't worry about how much of each type you're getting. A high-fiber diet can help prevent heart disease, cancer, high blood pressure, obesity, and diabetes (Anderson 1990).

Other good sources of fiber are beans and legumes, rice bran, brown rice, nuts, broccoli, oranges, and bran. Sonia has written a cookbook called *A World of Choices* (Gaemi 1990), and has developed a supplement that uses fiber and essential fats to help balance the body's blood-sugar levels and reduce cravings. For more information, visit Sonia's Web site at www.drsonia.com.

As a good rule of thumb, try to limit your intake of high-glycemic and "white" processed foods high in sugar and hydrogenated fats like pastries, cookies, white bread, potatoes, white rice, and chips. Look for dark-colored foods like whole-grain pasta, soba noodles, buckwheat, whole-grain seeded or sprouted-wheat breads, sprouted garbanzos, lentils, hummus, amaranth, kamut, and brown rice. (See our discussion of the glycemic index earlier in this chapter.)

Complex carbohydrates, phytohormonal foods, and high-fiber foods balance your insulin levels, reduce cravings, and help satisfy your appetite for a longer time than simple carbohydrates do. A diet high in these elements helps keep your moods balanced by keeping your neurotransmitters functioning properly, and also helps your body to remain hydrated. Foods high in fiber and complex carbs are generally inexpensive, easy-to-prepare foods that can be cooked in many different satisfying ways. In some parts of the world, it's estimated that 70 to 80 percent of peoples' food intake is made up of fiber-rich complex carbohydrates. Sonia's Antioxidant Smoothie is a recipe that offers sweetness as well as complex carbs.

BONE FOOD

Everyone should pay attention to their bone health, especially women, who may start to lose bone density as they age (Riggs and Melton 1992). Bone health also depends on staying active and well hydrated. Pregnant women need to pay special attention to their bone health and make sure they get enough calcium, but all women over thirty-five should take care to get enough calcium, through foods as well as supplements.

Many vegetables, especially leafy greens like kale, arugula, dandelion greens, watercress, and mustard greens, contain boron, magnesium, potassium, vitamin D, vitamin K, and zinc, which are necessary for healthy calcium absorption. Hummus, almonds,

This smoothie was designed to be an excellent source of antioxidants. Eat this 1-3 times daily, at any meal or as a snack. Blended fruits are preferable to juice in this smoothie, as the skin, peel, and pulp are rich in phytohormones and fibers. Makes 2-3 smoothies. (Can be stored in the refrigerator for 3-4 days.) Ingredients are as follows:

- **4 coddled eggs or egg whites (see directions below), ½ cup egg substitute, or 2 tsp. dried egg powder**

- **1 tbsp. roasted garbanzo flour**

- **1 tbsp. soy flour, buckwheat flour, or amaranth flour**

- **¼ cup soft tofu, ½ cup organic, low-fat plain yogurt or ½ cup soy milk, almond milk, or a combination**

- **2 tbsp. rice bran**

- **¼ cup sprouted garbanzos or red-colored sprouts (optional)**

- **1-3 tbsp. ground flaxseeds**

- **1 tsp. honey or stevia (optional)**

- **¼ cup frozen unsweetened cranberry juice concentrate or raisins (optional)**

- **Pinch of nutmeg, cardamom, ginger, rose hips, cumin, cinnamon, or powdered or chopped licorice root**

- **1 cup fresh, frozen, or dried berries of your choice (no strawberries)**

- **1 cup papaya, cantaloupe, watercress, and/or cilantro (optional)**

- **Fresh mint sprig, cinnamon stick, or pinch of chocolate as a garnish**

Combine all ingredients and blend for 3 minutes in a blender, adjusting the ingredients to the desired consistency. Serve immediately. Refrigerate any unused portion for future snacks or meals. You can even substitute a smoothie for ice cream or other high-fat desserts.

* **To coddle eggs:** *Coddle whole eggs in their shells by placing them in boiling water for 50 seconds. Peel or crack the eggs and add to the smoothie. You can cook several eggs at once and store them in the refrigerator for up to one week. Mark the shells so you can tell which eggs are coddled and which are not. If you prefer hard-boiled egg whites, cook the eggs longer and use the whites only. If not using the yolks, separate and save them for another use, such as for pets or as a sandwich filling.*

culinary herbs, rice bran, flaxseeds, sprouts, tofu, beets, soft cheeses such as feta, cottage cheese, and ricotta, and organic yogurt fortified with vitamin D are also good foods for bones.

Use your food journal to make sure you eat foods high in the elements needed to absorb calcium, as well as ensuring that you get some physical activity every day, get enough physical and mental rest, drink enough water and tea, and get enough sunlight (with proper sun protection, of course).

Yogurt: The Miracle Food

Yogurt is an ancient healing food that's been used all over the world. It's great for bone health and can be a wonderful base for mixing spices, herbs, nuts, flowers, flaxseeds, and fruit to satisfy any taste. It's used in dips, soups, salad dressing, sauces, and cereal. Yogurt is a good source of protein and is high in calcium, vitamin K, and magnesium. When it contains live cultures, it encourages the growth of helpful bacteria in your intestines. It enhances your natural digestive enzymes and helps to balance hormones. Eat yogurt with live cultures as often as you wish, but especially if you are taking antibiotic medications or if you suffer from irritable bowel syndrome or other problems with your digestive system. Yogurt can also help balance your hormones (especially estrogen, insulin, and progestin), strengthen your immune system, and calm your mind, and the calcium in yogurt may help with weight loss. We recommend eating organic unflavored yogurt fortified with vitamin D and adding your own flavors.

SUPPLEMENTS AND ENZYMES

Although it's best to get your nutrients from foods rather than capsules, supplements can be an important part of eating hormonally, if used moderately and wisely. But everyone has different supplementation needs. Taking too many supplements, or the wrong kind, can be dangerous because supplements are not regulated by the government. Consult your physician, registered dietitian, nutritionist, or other health professional about the supplements and dosages that make the most sense for you.

Enzymes

Digestion and absorption begins in the mouth with enzymes released in the saliva by the action of chewing. It continues as food travels through the gut and is broken down into its biochemical constituents. Millions of chemical reactions occur as digestive bacteria and pancreatic enzymes break down the chemical components of food. Eating hormonally will help keep your body's enzymes in balance, especially if you include yogurt, apple cider vinegar, greens, sprouts, herbs, and spices as a regular part of your diet.

Enzyme supplements can help the digestive process, especially if your natural intestinal flora are out of balance due to illness, medications, an unhealthy diet, too much processed food, or stress. Irritable bowel syndrome begins with inflammation of the intestines and can be healed by rebalancing the acids and good digestive enzymes in the intestines. Remember, your dosage of enzyme supplements will depend on your specific needs, so it's best to consult a registered dietitian or health practitioner. You can also try the Enzyme-Boosting Tea to calm and balance your digestive system. ❧

Enzyme-Boosting Tea

This makes 1 cup of dry mix. Use 1 tbsp. of dry mix per cup of hot water after each meal.

- **½ cup mint or spearmint leaves**
- **1 tbsp. each of mugwort, mint, orange peel, fennel seeds, cardamom, and licorice powder**
- **1 tsp. crystal sugar, honey, or licorice root**

Variations: *A similar tea can also be made by pouring hot water over 1 black tea bag and adding 1 tsp. cardamom or mugwort and 1 tsp. honey to the hot water. Or mix it with Healthy & Wise Tea or Denna's Rooibos Chai.*

your personal food wisdom pyramid

Now you can create a pyramid of your own favorite foods. Use the foods listed on this pyramid and in your food collage as your basic menu plan. Food should please all your senses, not just taste, and what you enjoy eating may differ from what someone else enjoys. It's important to feed your senses based on your own likes and dislikes. Think of the bright colors of fresh greens, vegetables, and fruit; the satisfying crunch of fresh peppers; the smooth, creamy texture of yogurt; or the smell of a hearty tomato sauce, comforting tea, or a spicy bean soup—food can please all of your senses at once.

Start by listing your favorite foods in the categories below. When you're done, add these foods to the blank pyramid at the end of this chapter. Make a copy and post it somewhere in your kitchen where you'll see it often. When you shop, bring this list or the pyramid with you and buy at least two things from each category. When you feel you would like a change, add different items of different colors from charts or recipes you'll find later in this book.

When you eat, focus on the appearance, smell, texture, and taste of the foods in front of you. Breathe in the aroma deeply, and exhale slowly. Eating slowly and mindfully helps your body feel full faster, since there is often a delay between the time your stomach is full and the moment your brain get the message that you're full and tells you to stop eating. Remember, eating hormonally should not mean eating bland, boring food that leaves you unsatisfied after your meal. Eat food that you enjoy eating. People who diet or otherwise restrict their eating so they feel unsatisfied may binge on junk foods or other satisfying, high-fat foods because they feel deprived.

YOUR PERSONAL SHOPPING LIST

Start by listing as many of your favorite foods as possible in each category, looking at your collage for inspiration. Try to add as many colors and varieties as you can think of, concentrating on the foods we recommend in this book. Remember to focus on foods that are rated low or medium on the glycemic index (discussed earlier in this chapter). Use your food diary to experiment with different kinds of foods until you find those you like. Expand your culinary horizons, and remember to experiment with different colors, textures, aromas, and tastes. Now, for each of the food categories below, begin listing the items you will include for your personal shopping list.

Tea

Tea can be a powerful healing food because it's so easy to adapt it to your particular health and wellness goals. Try green tea, black tea, rooibos, chai, and herbal teas. (Try Peaceful & Happy Tea, found earlier in this chapter.) Try using herbs, spices, dried berries, seeds, and flowers in your tea, as well.

_____

_____

_____

_____

Whole Grains (Bread, Pasta, Cereal, and Rice)

Examples: Barley; brown, black, and wild rice; oats; millet; rye; quinoa; amaranth; buckwheat; spelt; bran; long-grained rice; whole-grain bread; whole wheat pasta; soba or buckwheat noodles; sprouted grains.

_____

_____

_____

_____

Vegetables, Greens, Herbs, and Spices

All foods in this category are delicious as colorful main meals or side dishes and make easy, tasty snacks that please all your senses. Greens can include spinach, arugula, kale, dandelion greens, bitter melon, baby lettuce, watercress, seaweed, or purslane; vegetables can include broccoli, cauliflower, leeks, carrots, radishes, turnips, bok choy, squash, tomatoes, green beans, radish, daikon, peppers, and avocado.

Some culinary herbs are oregano, chives, parsley, cilantro, mint, tarragon, rosemary, basil, dill, garlic, ginger, sage, or marjoram. Spices include turmeric, cayenne, licorice root, cinnamon, cloves, pepper, and fenugreek.

_____

_____

_____

_____

Fruits

Choose fruits that are not too soft. If they are not ripe when you buy them, they can be ripened on a windowsill or in a brown paper bag. Fruits include pears, Asian pears, papayas, raspberries, apples, oranges, bananas, tangerines, grapes, plums, peaches, cantaloupe, grapefruit, watermelon, dates, figs, pomegranates, guavas, blueberries, blackberries, nectarines, cherries, kiwis, lemons, pineapple, limes, persimmons, and dried fruits like berries, apricots, papaya, or figs (without added sugar or sulfites). Remember to bring home as many colors as you can.

_____

_____

_____

_____

Beans, Legumes, Seeds, Nuts, and Sprouts

Examples: Garbanzo beans, soybeans, tofu, hummus, lentils, peas, black beans, peanuts, almonds, walnuts, flaxseeds, pumpkin seeds, and black sesame seeds. Also, try sprouts made from soybeans, garbanzo beans, mung beans, wheat berries, and alfalfa, red clover, radish, and daikon seeds.

Bone Foods

Bone foods are high in protein and calcium. These include feta, ricotta, and cottage cheese; tofu; hummus; soy milk; yogurt; seaweed; almond milk; buttermilk; and eggs. Leafy greens and culinary herbs are also considered bone foods (see Vegetables, Greens, Herbs, and Spices in this section.) You can use hard cheeses such as cheddar, jack, and Swiss cheese, but remember to use them sparingly, as flavoring for the dish rather as a main component.

Phosphorous foods can limit your body's ability to absorb calcium. If you are at risk for osteoporosis or other diseases that affect the bones, try to limit your intake of high-phosphorous foods such as soda, beer, and chocolate.

Meat, Fish, and Poultry

Eating hormonally means, with the exception of yogurt, eggs, certain cheeses, and some fish, restricting your intake of animal foods. If you still want to enjoy meat, try to eat leaner cuts and use small portions to flavor dishes made up of plant foods. Suggestions for this category of the pyramid include salmon, eggs, tuna, and organically raised chicken and turkey. Eat fish such as wild-caught salmon, trout, and chunk light tuna packed in water two to three times a week for excellent sources of essential fatty acids and protein.

Salt, Sugar, and Oils

Use salt, sugar, and oils sparingly, but remember that it's important to enjoy your food, so give yourself a treat occasionally. Olive oil is healthy for cooking, although be sure to keep the heat at medium, since olive oil overheats at a lower temperature than other oils. Olive oil is also good in dressings and sauces. Flax, walnut, and sesame oils are great cold as salad dressings and over pasta.

You can also use flavored vinegars, like balsamic or rice vinegar, to flavor dishes instead of or in addition to oil. You will use less oil and the dish will be more flavorful. Avoid using margarine and spreads made from hydrogenated oils. It's healthier to use a small amount of real butter than to use margarine.

Try to use herbs and spices more than sugar and salt to flavor your food, and challenge yourself to find healthful sweets such as date rolls, berries, red grapes, natural licorice or ginger candy, or fruit-and-nut candies. Try the Heart-Healthy Spice Mix (see the recipe earlier in this chapter) instead of salt. Fruit puree, dates, raisins, berries, honey, candy made with licorice root, stevia, and blackstrap molasses make great natural sweeteners. Limit your use of processed white sugar, most commercial packaged foods, and diet foods, and avoid artificial sweeteners.

_____

_____

❧

your personal food pyramid

Now, list your food choices on the blank pyramid on the next page and post it in a place where you will see it every day.

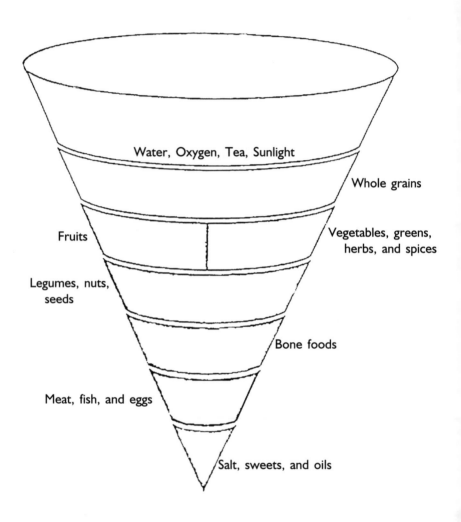

Water, Oxygen, Tea, Sunlight

Whole grains

Fruits

Vegetables, greens,
herbs, and spices

Legumes, nuts,
seeds

Bone foods

Meat, fish, and eggs

Salt, sweets, and oils

Your Personal Food Wisdom Pyramid

chapter 2

become your own food and lifestyle coach

There are more reasons to eat than simply satisfying your hunger. Food can heal your body, and enjoying food can heal your mind. Sharing food with friends and family makes us feel connected and balanced, and should be a vital part of everyone's life. Giving food—cooking meals for friends, making food to give as gifts, sharing recipes with neighbors—brings joy to the giver as well as the recipient and strengthens your connection with others.

One useful way to begin a lifetime of eating hormonally is to explore your specific needs and decide what you want to accomplish with your new lifestyle. Or you may have particular symptoms you want to heal. Are you lethargic, depressed, or tired much of the time? Do you want to lose or gain weight? Are you pregnant or nursing? Do you have a chronic health problem like diabetes, depression, high blood pressure, or high cholesterol that you want to manage better? Perhaps you have an autoimmune disease like multiple sclerosis or lupus. Are you fighting a life-threatening illness like cancer, osteoporosis, or heart disease? Every one of these health issues will affect what foods you should eat. Keeping a journal allows you to explore these issues in depth and then to make changes for the better.

For example, Willow, a client of Sonia's, used her journal to help discover why she was experiencing weight problems, food cravings, dizziness, anxiety, and mood swings. ❧

Willow's story

When Willow couldn't lose weight, even though she was obsessively sticking to a strict nonfat diet, she came to Dr. Sonia's Food Wisdom Therapy Clinic. Willow didn't know that essential fats are necessary to balance metabolism as well as neurotransmitters and hormones. In addition to essential fats, Willow's diet lacked fiber and phytohormonal foods because she mainly ate simple carbohydrates and foods high on the glycemic index (see chapter 1), which she craved because she was undernourished. Even though she ate no fats, she continued gaining weight from the many empty calories in the starches and sugars she was eating.

She was forty-four, and experiencing hot flashes, mood swings, and fatigue, which she thought of as normal for a woman of her age. Willow didn't know that these (and other symptoms of hormonal changes) may be influenced by the fluctuation of blood sugar. Her diet of simple carbohydrates caused her body's insulin levels to be constantly out of balance, and when her blood-sugar level dropped, she felt shaky and tired, and experienced headaches, anxiety, mood swings, and food cravings. Her lack of essential nutrients exacerbated her premenopausal symptoms, and the resulting hormonal imbalance may have contributed to her weight gain.

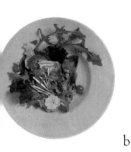

Sonia suggested to Willow that she should track her foods and their colors in her food journal and begin eating hormonally by increasing the amounts of fiber-rich and phytohormonal foods in her diet, foods such as roasted and sprouted garbanzo beans, beets, greens, wheat germ, rice bran, dried berries and dates, flax and fennel seeds, and teas like Healthy & Wise Tea and Denna's Rooibos Chai. Willow's challenge was to change her eating habits, from quick-fix, processed sweets and simple carbohydrates to therapeutic, nutritious cooked foods including lots of herbs, greens, fruits, tea, yogurt, and garbanzos. Willow also began writing positive thoughts in her journal every day.

Throughout the day, Willow needed to eat six small, frequent meals made of medium- and low-glycemic foods (see chapter 1) to balance her blood sugar and to eliminate her mood swings and other symptoms of low blood sugar. Sonia taught her some simple acupressure healing exercises to help her organs absorb the nutrients in her food more efficiently, and Willow began taking wheat germ oil capsules, enzyme supplements, and organic multivitamins that provided her the recommended dietary allowance (RDA) of magnesium, folic acid, vitamin B, calcium, and chromium.

In her journal, Willow set small daily goals for herself, starting by following the Eating Hormonally Cleansing Plan three days a week (see chapter 3). She began eating a lunch every day of a leafy green salad with sprouts, flaxseeds, walnuts, berries, and tofu or feta cheese, with organic low-fat yogurt, and a bowl of miso, vegetable, or lentil soup (see chapter 3). Then she increased her nutritious meals until she was eating hormonally most of the time. She ate fresh vegetables, fruits, grains, legumes, yogurt, feta cheese, eggs, and other healthful foods, including fish two to three times a week. Sonia explained to her that blood-sugar levels change hormone levels, and that eating small meals and frequent snacking on fiber

Denna's Rooibos Chai

A cupful of Denna's Rooibos Chai uses the refreshing taste of the South African rooibos plant, a sweet herb full of antioxidants. This delightful mixture blends the zing of pepper and allspice with the sweetness of nutmeg, ginger, and licorice. It balances the body's acidity and alkalinity and can help reduce cravings. Caffeine-free, Rooibos Chai is great as a latte, with soy or almond milk.

Combine 1 tbsp. of each ingredient:

Ginger (minced fresh or powdered)

Rooibos tea

Powdered or chopped licorice root

Orange peel

Cardamon

Add ½ tbsp. of the following mix: cayenne pepper; black pepper; fennel; coriander; nutmeg; allspice; cinnamon; rose hips

Mix 1-2 tbsp. of the tea mixture in ½ a cup of hot water, then add soy milk or more hot water.

keep blood sugar stable and insulin balanced, which, in turn, balances mood and keeps the body working well.

Keeping a journal allowed Willow to make lifestyle changes that gave her more energy, balanced moods, an end to hot flashes and headaches, and she began to lose weight. She also bought a meditation tape, and a videotape of qi gong and self-acupressure. She learned easy techniques to increase the energy flow throughout her body and mind, and to help her body cleanse itself of toxins. Today, she has the tools to cope with stress and anxiety. She's enjoyed becoming her own lifestyle coach, and now, whenever she can, she enjoys physical exercise, "quiet-mind" time, self-acupressure, and deep breathing. Here's the recipe Willow used to make her tea. 🥀

your healing and wellness goals

This food journal will help you meet your healing and wellness goals. To begin, you must figure out what your goals are. Use the following exercise to clarify what you hope to accomplish by working with this book.

YOUR PHYSICAL HEALTH

Are you premenopausal, menopausal, or postmenopausal or experiencing other hormonal changes?

Do you suffer from PMS?

Do you experience hot flashes, night sweats, or insomnia?

Do you have an eating disorder?

Are you on hormone replacement therapy (HRT)?

Are you pregnant?

Nursing?

Are you overweight?

    How long have you been overweight?

Are you underweight?

    How long have you been underweight?

How much weight would you like to gain or lose per week?

Do you have troubling symptoms that come on suddenly, such as constipation, bloating, diarrhea, headaches, fatigue, indigestion, or cramps? List them below:

_____

_____

_____

_____

Do you have chronic health problems such as chronic pain with no apparent organic cause? Do you have diabetes, high blood pressure, recurring cancer, osteoporosis, skin problems, food intolerance, an autoimmune disorder, irritable bowel syndrome, or depression or other mood imbalances? If so, list them below:

_____

_____

_____

_____

_____

Do you often have unpleasant food-related symptoms, such as gas or abdominal pain, fatigue, jitteriness, anxiety, or a mood change after eating? Describe the situations that cause you to experience food-related symptoms (e.g., after you eat spicy foods, you have painful gas).

_____

_____

_____

_____

_____

Working with this journal will help you discover patterns in your food-related symptoms. If you are allergic or sensitive to any particular foods, you can find tasteful substitutes by testing new food choices and noting how they make you feel. This journal and Sonia's earlier book, *Eating Wisely for Hormonal Balance* (Gaemi 2004), will help you find foods that can heal or alleviate conditions such as weight problems, diabetes, depression, arthritis, menopausal hot flashes, PMS, or symptoms related to pre- or postmenopause. You can visit Sonia's Web site at www.drsonia.com. Even if you suffer from a chronic condition like arthritis, you may be able to lessen your discomfort and support healing your body by eating hormonally.

YOUR EMOTIONAL WELLNESS

Physical health is important, but emotional health is just as important. Our emotional states are linked to our physical health in ways still being studied, but high levels of depression, stress, or anxiety are thought to be directly linked to changes in immune functioning and increased susceptibility to certain diseases (Maier and Laudenslager 1985). Life, like food, is meant to be enjoyed, and even small changes in food and lifestyle can help you stay mentally and emotionally healthy and joyful.

Now, describe what you usually eat at each meal on an average day, and rate your enjoyment and energy level during the meal on a scale of 0 to 10, with 10 as your optimum state. Think about the taste, aroma, color, and appearance of the food, its healthfulness, how much time you take to eat, whether you feel tired and lethargic or energetic and alert, how you feel after you've eaten, and whether you take time away from other tasks to concentrate on your meal. Do you usually rush out of the house without sitting down for breakfast? Do you eat lunch at your desk while you work? Or do you greet the day by sitting down to eat a good, healthful breakfast, and take the time at lunch to visit a park or garden and get some sun? When you eat lunch, do you have trouble concentrating or do you feel sleepy? Or do you feel full of energy as you take a much-needed break with an invigorating walk, followed by a delicious and healthful meal before tackling your work again?

Breakfast: _____

_____

_____

Enjoyment and energy level: _____

Late morning snack: _____

_____

Enjoyment and energy level: _____

Lunch: _____

_____

_____

Enjoyment and energy level: _____

Afternoon snack: _____

_____

Enjoyment and energy level: _____

Dinner: _____

_____

Enjoyment and energy level: _____

Do you regularly have food cravings? What types of food do you crave and when does this happen (e.g., after eating your normal meal, or after eating a certain food)?

_____

_____

How would you like your average meals to change? Do you wish you had more time to enjoy your food, that you had more energy to create new and different meals, that you regularly ate healthier food, that you dined with your friends and family more often, or that you had the time to try out new recipes? Here, you should list the things you would like to change about your average meals:

_____

_____

_____

_____

_____

Why haven't you made these changes until now? Reasons may include lack of knowledge about healthful eating, limited time to try out new recipes, too much work to go outdoors at lunch, lack of energy or motivation, or your family's resistance to trying new foods.

_____

_____

_____

_____

Now, think of ways in which you can make at least one meal a week be the joyful, mindful, fulfilling meal you would like all your meals to be. Take one of the reasons you listed above and write down a solution. For example, if you've thought that you don't know enough about food to cook healthy meals for yourself, one solution might be to try out some of the recipes in this book. If you have so much work to do that you think you can't take an hour, or even thirty minutes, to go outdoors at lunch and take your mind off work, one solution might be to start leaving work at lunchtime one day a week for a fifteen-minute break. If you eat lunch at your desk and spend your whole day feeling tense and anxious, one possible change might be to give yourself five minutes a day to do a qi gong or yoga movement or a deep breathing exercise with the office door closed.

Now, in the space provided, describe one action you can take in the next week to improve your eating patterns:

_____

_____

_____

_____

_____

_____

_____

As you use this food journal, use the information you've compiled here, as well as the recipes in this book, to make at least one meal a week a 9 or 10 on your enjoyment scale. As you get better at creating one simple, joyful meal a week, make it two meals a week, and then three, until you enjoy most of your meals. Enjoyment can mean that the meal is healthful, fast, tasty, and a treat for your senses, that you cook and dine with friends or family and share each others' healthy recipes, or that you take time to enjoy your meal with all of your senses, putting work or troubles aside for length of the meal. Ideally, you will experience all of these types of enjoyment in your meals. Make each meal a ritual of pleasure for all your senses and you will notice a change in your mind and body. ❧

planning your shopping trips

Eating hormonally is all about being aware enough to plan ahead for what your body and mind need to stay healthy and energetic. Many of us lead such busy lives that we can't imagine taking the time or having the energy to shop for new and healthy foods or to experiment with new recipes. It's all we can do to sit down for a meal at all. But planning and shopping for healthy food need not take more time than the shopping you already do. In fact, being tired, sick, or depressed often takes as much or more time out of your day as shopping for healthful foods would. Moreover, buying vibrant, delicious, colorful foods is much more fun.

When you constructed your personal Food Wisdom Pyramid, as instructed in chapter 1, you made a basic shopping list. Remember to buy at least two items of different colors from each section of the list each time you go shopping. In time, you may tire of buying the same foods on shopping trips. As you read and use this journal, take note of the recipes and ideas scattered throughout. If something looks good to you, copy the ingredients immediately and post your note where you put your shopping lists. As you find foods and recipes you enjoy, add those ingredients to your pyramid. Soon you'll have a master list of colorful, tasty, healthy foods that you can take with you whenever you buy groceries. You'll never come back from the grocery store with nothing but frozen pizza, cheddar cheese, snack crackers, and soda again.

SNACKS

Here's a way to make sure you snack on healthy foods during the day: Before you leave the house in the morning, gather small containers of dry tea, hummus and yogurt or feta cheese, foods such as cauliflower, avocado, carrots, Asian pear, almonds or other nuts, and a slice or two of whole wheat bread. This will give you all the nutrients you'll need all day. Eat the yogurt, fruit, and nuts, drink the tea, and dip the vegetables and bread in the hummus and yogurt for tasty, healthful snacks all day long.

Alternatives to Supermarkets

You needn't always shop at supermarkets, where a diverse selection of produce, spices, and herbs can be hard to come by. Here are some other places to get your favorite new foods:

Community supported farms: Why not have organic fruits and vegetables delivered to your home or office? Ask at your local farmer's market or health food co-op, look in the phone book, or check online at www.csacenter.org for local farms that will deliver. These farms often send recipes along with their produce. Some even let you choose the specific fruits and vegetables you want, and may even let you order nonproduce items like soy milk, organic chocolate and coffee, fruit juices, tea, pasta, bread, and sometimes even meat and fish. Many of these farms welcome visitors, which can make for a great day trip.

Farmer's markets: These have become weekly events in many parts of the country, and they're a great source of locally grown produce, as well as breads, honey, flowers, and other items. By buying at a local farmer's market, you support local growers and you know that your food hasn't traveled across the country to get to you.

Multicultural markets: If your community has neighborhoods where people from different cultures live, visit their markets. It can be like traveling to another country, without the expense of the plane fare. You can often find food items in these markets that you can't find at your local markets. Experiment by buying one or two unfamiliar items and challenge yourself to find ways to use them. Or ask a local shopper how to use the item, and become part of a mini multicultural exchange program.

The Internet: You can buy almost anything online. If there are hard-to-find items that you'd like to try, log on and order them from one of the thousands of independently owned shops on the Internet. Visit www.drsonia.com for more recipes and tips on using unfamiliar foods.

SOME SHOPPING AND KITCHEN TIPS

- Plan at least two meals for the week. These can be as simple as a smoothie one morning and an omelet the next, or as complicated as cooking a stuffed salmon with buckwheat pilaf for your cooking group and a mushroom-barley soup to eat all week. Add the ingredients to your shopping list. This way you know you'll have the ingredients on hand.

- Choose one item and figure out many different ways to use it in your cooking. For example, how many ways can you use garbanzo beans? Try adding them to soup, making hummus, sprouting them (see chapter 1 for instructions), sprinkling canned or sprouted garbanzos on your salads, and stir-frying sprouted garbanzos in olive oil with fresh sage and chopped red onion.

- If you don't have a spice and herb collection already, try to buy one spice and one dried herb, such as turmeric and dried dill, or powdered cayenne pepper and dried rosemary, each time you shop. This way, you'll wind up with great collection of herbs and spices for any meal you want to cook. Be sure to buy fresh herbs, such as basil and mint, for meals planned in advance.

  Tip: Fresh herbs kept in a glass of water or rolled in a damp paper towel in the refrigerator last longer. Also, if you grow your own, you'll always have fresh herbs handy.

- Go shopping with a friend. Remember to eat before you shop, so you won't be hungry in the store. Try different foods and treats, have tea together and make a ritual out of it, or make a picnic of some of the items you've bought. Make shopping day fun.

- Give each week a specific "theme." For example, one week you could decide to use Chinese recipes and buy water chestnuts, sprouts, ginger, snow peas, cabbage, lemongrass, dried chiles, and tofu.

- When you decide on recipes to cook for a week, consider doubling the recipe amounts so you'll have leftovers, or "encore meals." Freeze the leftovers to eat later or share with a friend. Start a cooking group where you and several friends get together to shop and cook. Choose a type of regional cuisine for that evening, such as Italian or Thai. Find recipes on the Internet, in cookbooks, or by visiting a local food store that carries food from that region. When the meal is ready, sit together and enjoy the aroma, textures, and tastes of the food as well as the pleasure of cooking and being together.

SAMPLE MENU FOR EATING HORMONALLY

Here's a sample menu for the eating hormonally plan. As you can see, this plan is not about restricting your food choices, but about eating nutritionally dense foods with a variety of colors, textures, and tastes that provide fiber, protein, phytohormones, antioxidants, minerals, and other nutrients to your body and balance your body's acidity and alkalinity. Remember, this is only a sample menu; what you eat will depend on your likes and dislikes, your lifestyle, and your healing goals. Several times a day, before you start your meals, take the time to take several deep, long inhales, and to empty your lungs completely on each exhale. If you wish, do a two to three minute gentle seated meditation before you get out of bed in the morning and before you go to sleep at night, focusing on the positives in your life. Consider following the cleansing plan (see chapter 3) several days a week.

Breakfast

- *Start with a pear and a glass of water or tea*

- *1-2 slices toasted bread (sprouted wheat, buckwheat, amaranth, garbanzo flour, whole-grain, rye, seeded, etc.) with feta cheese, tahini, or almond butter*

- *½ cup brown rice or other whole-grain cereal with berries or other fruits, in soy or almond milk or yogurt*

- *½ cup yogurt with seeds, nuts, or fruits*

- *1 cup of Denna's Rooibos Chai*

Morning Snack

- *Asian pear or apple slices (try wrapping them in seaweed sheets)*

- *1 cup of the tea of your choice, or coffee if you wish*

Lunch

- *Salad of spinach and arugula, with a few cubes of tofu, avocado, walnuts, black sesame seeds, and cubed roasted beets with a vinaigrette of olive oil and balsamic vinegar mixed with 2 tablespoons of yogurt and a few pinches of parmesan cheese*

- *Vegetarian or fish burrito without cheddar or other hard cheese*

- *Miso soup or vegetable and bean soup*

- *1 cup of the tea of your choice*

- *Natural ginger candy, date rolls, or fruit for dessert*

Afternoon Snack

- *7-9 (each) roasted almonds and dried cranberries or raisins*

- *½ cup of yogurt with fruit, honey, rose petals, or crystallized ginger*

- *1 cup of Healthy & Wise Tea*

Dinner

- *Medium-sized salad of mixed greens with feta cheese, walnuts, and a dressing of olive oil and balsamic vinegar*

- *3-ounce piece of wild-caught salmon, baked with sage, on a bed of wild rice cooked in miso broth*

- *1 cup of Peaceful & Happy Tea*

After-Dinner Snack

- *1 cup of melon slices from a variety of types of melon*

- *1 cup of chamomile tea or Peaceful & Happy Tea, to help you relax before bed*

Eating wisely doesn't mean eating boring foods or taking extra time out of every day to prepare lavish meals. Most of the foods discussed in this book are readily available at any well-stocked market. Now that you have some idea of your food goals, that is, whether to enjoy your meals more, to combat specific physical symptoms, to cope better with chronic problems, to lose or gain weight, to balance the body and mind, or to stop snacking on junk food, this journal will help you explore how eating hormonally can change your life.

chapter 3

using your food journal to become your own lifestyle coach

Nobody can tell you how to eat and live; you are the only one who can decide which foods, exercises, and lifestyle choices are right for you. That's why the journal pages in chapter 4 are the heart and soul of this book. Use your journal to track your physical and emotional states so you can begin making informed choices, not only about the foods and liquids you consume, but also how much physical movement, breathing, and "quiet mind" time you do in a day. In this chapter, we'll examine the categories you'll see in the journal pages, and provide an overview of how to track your days. We'll discuss how to analyze these categories, and give suggestions for ways to look at each aspect of your life. Your journal entries will help you to become your own self-healing lifestyle coach.

keep a journal for a healthy body and mind

People who are trying to slim down tend to lose more weight and to keep it off longer when they track their eating and exercise patterns in a journal. Similarly, research has proven that people who've experienced trauma or loss or are having emotional problems like depression or anxiety also benefit from journal writing. People with chronic health problems visit the doctor less often when they use a journal, and patients with terminal illnesses experience less depression and stress if they describe their feelings in a diary (Pennebaker 2003). Sonia has found a food journal to be essential to her clients healing. ❧

Andrew's story

Andrew, a college sophomore, suffered from stomach pains regularly followed by diarrhea. The campus doctor diagnosed stress-related irritable bowel syndrome and prescribed an antianxiety drug. Andrew did have a very busy schedule—a full class load, a part-time job, and a girlfriend, and sometimes he did feel stressed-out and anxious, but he usually dealt with this by taking a brisk run through campus.

That same week, the controversy surrounding antianxiety and antidepressant drugs was being discussed in his psychology class, so he was reluctant to take a drug. He'd seen Sonia's TV show, *The Art of Self-Healing with Dr. Sonia*, in his nutrition class one day, in which she'd discussed keeping a food journal. So, instead of filling his prescription for the antianxiety medication, he chose to keep a food journal to find out what, exactly, was causing his stomach problems.

He recognized that, if he tracked his meals, moods, and goals, he would learn to see himself, his body, and what he ate as an interconnected whole. So he began to take note of what and when he ate, and when his stomach problems occurred.

Some time later, when he examined his journal he found that the stomachache had occurred three times the first week of taking notes: after a morning muffin with a latte; after a smoothie he'd made at home; and after eating an energy bar on his way to class one day. None of these foods had any common ingredients, except the latte and the smoothie, both of which included milk. Thinking he might be lactose-intolerant, he cut out all dairy products for a week. Unfortunately, his stomach upsets continued.

Then, he noticed that he had stomach pains about an hour after eating an energy bar, which he always ate between classes when he didn't have time to fix and eat a regular meal. Reviewing the ingredients of the energy bar, he noticed it contained isolated soy protein, or soy powder, which he also used in his homemade smoothies as a source of protein. He replaced the energy bars with a handful of almonds and an Asian pear, and his stomach problems lessened. On most days, though, he still had diarrhea. Looking through his journal entries, he realized the diarrhea occurred in the late morning, shortly after his daily latte. He wondered if he was sensitive to coffee and switched to an herbal tea.

Easy-to-make smoothies had been Andrew's breakfast staple. One morning, since it seemed that perhaps he wasn't lactose-intolerant, he made a smoothie without the soy powder, using a recipe he'd learned while watching Sonia's TV show. The recipe used yogurt, fresh fruit, hard-cooked egg whites for protein, honey, two tablespoons of psyllium husks for fiber, one tablespoon of turmeric, and a pinch of cardamom. That day he was very pleased not to have any stomach pain or diarrhea. After months of making entries in his food journal, Andrew finally tracked down the culprits: soy powder and coffee.

Many people don't know that too much soy can trigger food sensitivities because the soybeans grown in the United States often are bioengineered to include protein from the Brazil nut. Also, American soy products are often incorrectly fermented and not aged appropriately, so that the protein in the soy may cause allergic reactions in people who eat too much soy-based food, such as tofu, tempeh, and miso (Sevrens 2000). ❧

the food journal categories

In this section, we discuss the categories you'll be asked to track in your food journal. We've added suggestions, tips, and even recipes to these descriptions to give you ideas on how to use these categories to support your physical and mental health.

MOODS AND THOUGHTS ON WAKING

Often, your mood when you wake up can affect your entire day. This is why we ask you to track your moods. When you awake, pay attention to how you feel. Do you feel energetic, contented, and well-rested, or sluggish, depressed, or anxious? Stay in bed for a few minutes and track your thoughts. Are you worrying about a problem at work, anxious because of all you must do, or are you eager to start the day? Jot your thoughts down in the appropriate place on that day's food journal page.

Moods are not just emotional changes that we cannot control. They are often affected by external factors, such as what we eat and drink, how much exercise we get, our stress levels and hormonal balances, the chemicals our bodies secrete (such as endorphins and neurotransmitters), and environmental factors like chemicals, pollution, and the amount of sunlight we get.

By tracking our moods, we can learn how certain foods and other factors might affect us. For example, if you wake up lethargic and a little depressed some mornings but not others, you can use your food journal to discover whether you ate specific foods the day before that might be contributing to your low mood.

Do you feel depressed in the mornings after a night of drinking alcohol, smoking cigarettes, or eating too much? Does having a stressful day, eating fatty or starchy foods, not getting enough sleep, talking to a very negative person, or overindulging in sweets bring your mood down? Or you might notice that you feel lethargic and tired after eating dairy or wheat products, which may point to an allergy or food sensitivity.

If your journal indicates that certain foods seem to coincide with low moods, fatigue, or other unpleasant symptoms, then you can try cutting out that food or changing your habits for a week to see if it really is the culprit. In the case of a possible food sensitivity, spend several days cleansing using Sophia's Seeds Formula (the recipe appears later in this chapter) to help your body naturally detoxify. Then slowly reintroduce the foods you think you may be sensitive to. Eat yogurt (try organic goat-milk yogurt) daily and drink two to three cups of mint tea with honey or Denna's Rooibos Chai each day to help balance your body's acidity, hormones, and digestive enzymes. Try meditating, taking a relaxing walk, or doing breathing exercises throughout the day.

If you tend to wake up feeling anxious or stressed and there doesn't seem to be any link to your food, your lifestyle may be contributing to these difficult emotional states. Perhaps you need to set a time in the morning to do simple exercises to focus on your breathing, such as qi gong or yoga, to center yourself and start your day in a better mood. Maybe you need to take a short walk to calm yourself, or slow down for a few mindful minutes with a cup of comforting tea.

Chronic stress has been linked to depression, anxiety, chronic fatigue, obesity, diabetes, and an increased risk of serious physical health problems. If you feel stressed most of the time, consider making some lifestyle changes to lower your stress levels, as well as to experiment with techniques to cope with stress in a more productive way. Moderate regular exercise, time to quiet the mind, creative pursuits, interesting hobbies, and a fulfilling social life are all ways you can help yourself get breaks from stressful life circumstances. If stress is leading to depression, panic attacks, or the overuse of alcohol or drugs, group or individual therapy may be able to help.

MOVEMENT

Our bodies are designed to move, but in today's world more and more of us live sedentary lives. We sit in our offices all day and then drive anywhere we need to go. It's no surprise that obesity is a major public health concern in the U.S. This category of the food journal is called "movement" rather than "exercise" because "exercise" implies high-impact activity like jogging, aerobics, or weight training. But there are many movement options for creating good health other than high-impact activities.

Low-impact movement practices like yoga, tai chi, and qi gong not only strengthen your muscles and improve your breathing, balance, and stamina, they also ask you to enter a focused, meditative state, which can lower your stress and anxiety levels (Raub 2002), cholesterol (Wang, Collet, and Lau 2004), and blood pressure (Sancier 1999). They help balance the energy of the body and mind and have been used for thousands of years by people all over the world.

Walking is one of the best exercises (Slentz et al. 2004), and dancing, swimming, golfing, tennis, and gardening are other forms of movement that help your body as well as your mind. Jogging has an equal effect to Zoloft, the antidepressant medication, and it lasts a lot longer, but even brisk walking helps depressed people feel better (Servan-Schreiber 2004). Regular, moderate exercise improves the body's overall fitness and may protect against health problems such as coronary heart disease, hypertension, obesity, diabetes, osteoporosis, and certain cancers (Pate et al. 1995).

Try to get as much movement as you can into your day, and report this in your food journal. Take the stairs instead of the elevator when you can, and walk or bicycle to the corner store instead of driving. When you walk to the store, write down how many minutes you walked. If you did some yoga poses or qi gong movements, record those as well. If you take a break at lunch and just walk around the block or do some stretching at your desk, record this in your journal, and pay attention to how you feel on the days you get more movement and the days when you get less.

The amount of movement you need in a day depends on your personal goals. If you want to lose weight, more vigorous exercise combined with low-impact movement like yoga, qi gong, or walking will be necessary. When trying to lose body fat, take care not to eat one hour before or after any vigorous exercise or movement session (you may drink water, tea, or Sophia's Seeds Formula, however), and try to eat more frequent, smaller meals throughout the day rather than two or three large ones. Drink one to three cups of Healthy & Wise Tea daily (the recipe appears later in this chapter). If you are simply trying to maintain your normal weight, thirty to sixty minutes a day of moderate movement is usually enough to create and maintain good health and balanced energy.

As with your eating habits, you are likely to stick to an exercise or movement routine only if you enjoy it, so the type of movement you do is not as important as the fact that you do some kind of movement in the first place. Find a type of movement or exercise practice that you enjoy doing and makes you feel energized, then keep track of how and for how long you move your body every day. You may be surprised to discover that you're getting more movement than you thought you were.

MEDITATION AND CONSCIOUS BREATHING

Meditation is an ancient practice that uses breathing and mindfulness to quiet the mind and body and to open the heart to compassion. Meditating provides many health benefits, including strengthening the immune system (Davidson et al. 2003), lowering blood pressure (Wallace et al. 1983), reversing or preventing stress-related health problems (MacLean et al. 1997), and promoting better psychological and physical health in cancer patients (Carlson et al. 2004).

The mindfulness-based stress reduction method has been used successfully to treat depression, chronic pain, psoriasis, fibromyalgia, and anxiety. It is taught in several major hospitals. Even spending just five minutes a day quietly sitting in a peaceful place, taking deep breaths, and letting go of your day's worries can be beneficial. If it's hard to get time to yourself, set a goal of only ten minutes one day a week, then increase your "quiet mind" time to ten minutes a day, and then to fifteen or twenty minutes a day. Turn off the phone, the TV, and the computer, and sit in a place where you won't be disturbed. Just sit in a relaxed pose, gently focus on your breathing, and allow your mind to free itself from its day-to-day worries. To learn more about meditation, visit your local bookstore or library, visit www.drsonia.com, or check out meditation classes in your area.

Because breathing is a regular, unstoppable body function that's easy to track, meditation practices often ask you to focus on your breath as a way to shift your mind's attention away from your thoughts. Most of us take breathing for granted, as something our bodies just do naturally. But because most of us don't pay attention to our breathing, we breathe shallowly, not expanding our lungs fully when we inhale, or not expelling all the air from our lungs when we exhale. Shallow breathing can limit the body's oxygen intake, leading to fatigue, impairment of skeletal muscle and lung function, and exercise intolerance (Bernardi et al. 1998).

Breathe for Energy

Doing breathing exercises expands your lung capacity, which improves the flow of oxygen to all of your body systems and provides life-giving nutrients and energy. These exercises also are good ways to center your mind when you can't take time out to meditate or to get away from what's happening around you. You can do them anywhere; for example, while stuck in traffic in your car, as you wait on hold on the phone, or while standing in line at the bank. Here are two breathing exercises to get you started. Try to spend at least fifteen minutes a day doing deep breathing, and record in your journal how you feel as your body responds to the increased oxygen and the mental calm that accompanies conscious breathing.

Breathing for lung energy: This exercise clears the lungs, builds stamina, can help with weight loss, and builds up good digestive enzymes. Sit or stand in a comfortable position. Place your tongue gently on the roof of your mouth, just behind your top teeth. Through your nose, breathe in positive energy and life force to the count of four, filling up your lungs so your belly extends. Hold the air for five counts. Then exhale through your mouth, exhaling any negative energy you may be holding in your body, for ten counts. Do this for several cycles, and then return to normal breathing. Once you've practiced several times, increase the time you inhale to the count of eight, hold the air for eight counts, and then exhale to the count of sixteen, tightening your stomach muscles as you exhale to push all the air out of your lungs. The goal is to exhale for twice as long as you inhale. If you become dizzy, breathe normally until the dizziness passes.

Breathing for stress and tension reduction: To get rid of negative energies and the carbon dioxide in your body, do deep inhalations and exhalations to reach a state of relaxation. To begin, inhale through your nose, breathing in positive life force and energy, and fill your lungs with oxygen. As your lungs fill to capacity, your abdomen should expand. As you begin to slowly exhale, imagine the tension and negative energy in your body flowing out with your breath. Exhale for two or three times as long you inhaled, tightening your stomach muscles to get all the used air out of your lungs. Silently or aloud, say "My body is getting light. I am becoming one with the Earth." Repeat this exercise several times, focusing your attention on the tension and stress in all areas of your body, and with your mind's eye, watch as the stress flows out with your breath. Continue until you feel free of tension.

CLEANSING FOR HEALING AND ENERGY

As we live in this world, we accumulate toxins from the foods we eat, the pollution in the air and water, and from the byproducts of stress and anxiety. We also accumulate toxins from smoking, drinking, and taking medications or supplements, and from preservatives and other compounds in the manufactured products all around us. Many products and foods (including dairy and meat from animals treated with growth hormones), contain *xenoestrogens*, or artificially created compounds that have estrogen-like effects on our bodies. Xenoestrogens have been linked to breast cancer, pregnancy problems, weight fluctuations, early menopause, PMS, early onset of puberty, endometriosis, and other health problems, although the effects of xenoestrogens in humans are still being studied. The body is always in the process of cleansing itself, through the kidneys, gall bladder, and liver, and the following cleansing program was designed to boost your body's natural healing ability. Almost every culture in the world has a tradition of internal cleansing. Sonia has seen that following her rules for cleansing days helps her clients recover from health problems and gives them new energy.

The Food Wisdom Pyramid (see chapter 1) with its emphasis on organically grown whole grains, fresh fruits, vegetables, nuts, seeds, herbs, and spices, is already low in chemicals, pesticides, preservatives, and processed foods, but for an added boost, try using the Sophia's Seeds Formula (see below) to help your digestive system expel potentially poisonous toxins. This eating hormonally plan is the first program to introduce seeds as healing foods. The seeds in Sophia's Seeds Formula work by moving through the colon without being broken down by digestive juices. As they travel, they help push food waste through the intestines and out of the body. This cleansing plan will maintain health and keep you feeling and looking young. It's especially helpful if you are an athlete, want to lose weight, are trying to become pregnant, have PMS, are menopausal, have osteoporosis, or are healing from cancer.

You can choose to do a cleansing day once or twice a week or you can choose to eat this way every day. If, for example, you sometimes like to indulge in a rich meal, complete with a decadent dessert, you can take the day after as a cleansing day. It's up to you when to take a cleansing day (or days), but when you do take one, be sure to note it in your journal.

This is a powerful drink to aid your digestive system in eliminating waste and potential toxins from your intestines. This recipe uses 2¼ cups of whole seed mix, and makes enough for up to 9 servings or 9 days (¼ cup or 6 tbsp. per day). Flax, basil, and psyllium seeds are probably the easiest to find, and the others are readily available in Middle Eastern, Chinese, and Indian food stores. You can use all the seeds listed, or you can choose two or three types of seeds to get started. Organic seed is recommended. See www.drsonia.com for a list of resources.

1 ¼ cups khak shir seeds

¼ cup basil seeds

¼ cup psyllium seeds

¼ cup flaxseeds

¼ cup black sesame seeds

Mix the seeds and store them in a dry area.

Preparation and use: For individual servings, wash ¼ cup (or 6 tbsp.) of Sophia's Seeds Formula by rinsing them in a bowl and then pouring off the water. Mix the seeds with 2 cups of filtered water (if you prefer juice to water, use unsweetened cranberry, pomegranate, or another juice without any artificial sweetener). Mix the liquid and seeds together in a water bottle or other container (plastic is okay). Drink half of the mixture in the morning before eating, and drink the rest throughout the day. Or, drink half in the morning and the other half at night before eating. Or you can keep adding water to the bottle, sipping all day. In hot climates, keep the formula refrigerated.

Optional methods: Some of Sonia's clients prefer to put 1 tbsp. of seeds on their tongue and swallow them whole, followed by drinking two glasses of water. Or you can have 2 tbsp. of seed mixture before every meal. Be sure to follow this with two glasses of water. If you have trouble with whole seeds, you can use the seed husks instead. Another option is to add seeds to yogurt or pureed fruits, followed by two glasses of water. Caution: Swallowing seeds without water can cause constipation. If you have diverticulitis or other intestinal problems, whole seeds are not recommended.

If your journal shows you a pattern of sluggishness, fatigue, depression, unexplained weight gain or loss, mood swings, or other troubling symptoms, try two or three cleansing days to assess whether your body is responding to a buildup of toxins from rich foods, medication, drugs or alcohol, or other causes. Such cleansing days can become a ritual when you begin new projects, to celebrate accomplishments, or because you feel that you need the renewed energy that cleansing brings. **Caution:** If you have diverticulitis or any other disorder of the intestine, use ground seeds and consult your doctor before consuming whole seeds. Do not stop taking any prescription medication unless directed to do so by your prescribing physician.

Eating Hormonally while Cleansing

On your cleansing days, eat the foods listed below. Focus on colored foods, plant foods, seeds, yogurt, and tea. Limit most meat, starches, hard cheese (e.g., cheddar and jack), simple carbohydrates like pastries, potato chips, soda, white breads, artificial sweetners, hydrogenated fats, nicotine, alcohol, and caffeine.

- At least 3-5 cups of tea, with fresh or dried herbs (especially mint and sage), and flowers (rose petals, rose hips, hibiscus, and lemon verbena). Denna's Rooibos Chai or Healthy & Wise Tea are especially good for cleansing days. If you enjoy coffee, try diluting it by half with filtered water or tea.

- As much as you want of organic, fresh vegetables (especially cabbage, cauliflower, daikon, turnips, yams, beets, bitter melon, lettuce, endive, and seaweed).

- At least 5 medium servings (½ cup each) of fruits (especially assorted berries, citrus, grapes, melons, apples, and pears) per cleansing day.

- 8-10 cups a day of filtered water for your seed formula, teas, and just to drink by itself.

- At least 5 cups per day of leafy greens (assorted baby lettuce, kale, spinach, mustard, Swiss chard, and arugula), fresh herbs (oregano, sage, rosemary, thyme, parsley, cilantro, and chives). Add to your soups, salads, stews, or smoothies.

- As much as you want of sprouts of alfalfa, red clover, buckwheat, daikon, garbanzo, lentil, mung beans, soybeans, or snow peas. Add to smoothies, omelets, and sandwiches, or eat raw as snacks. Try sprinkling them with flavored vinegar.

- 1-3 cups of organic low-fat yogurt or goat's milk yogurt daily. Almond or sunflower seed milk, tofu, soy milk, and buttermilk. (Try diluting yogurt with mineral water and adding dried mint.)

- Hummus, tahini, seed and nut pastes and butters like almond, walnut, or pumpkin seed butter.

- 1-2 cups daily of grains, including brown rice, amaranth, buckwheat, and quinoa. (Try bread made of sprouted grains.)

- Legumes, beans (especially ½-1 cup daily of roasted, sprouted, or canned garbanzos). Try roasted beans as a snack, or sprouted seeds and beans in stews and soups.

- 3-4 tablespoons daily of flaxseeds and rice bran. Try sprinkling them in your cereal, soups, salads, or smoothies.

- Spices, including turmeric, fenugreek, cumin, and cardamom. Try 1-2 tablespoons of your favorite herbs or spices daily in your smoothie, soup, yogurt, or tea.

- 1-2 tablespoons daily of oils made from olives, sesame seeds, walnuts, or nuts in dressings or sauces.

- 3-4 ounces 2-3 times per week of wild-caught fish or several organic eggs per week. Try 3-6 egg whites daily in a smoothie or hard-boiled egg whites in your salads and sandwiches.

If you are doing one to two days of cleansing, eating eggs and fish is optional. But if you are eating this way every day, be sure to eat fish two to three times a week for the protein and omega-3 and omega-6 essential fatty acids.

Cleansing-Day Menu Plan

To give you some idea of how varied, colorful, and delicious your cleansing days can be, here is a sample cleansing-day menu plan. Be aware of your food choices and pay attention to your sensations and emotions when eating. These foods will leave you feeling alert, fresh, and energized and may help ease cravings for fatty, starchy, salty, or sweet foods, as well as for nicotine, caffeine, and alcohol.

Breakfast: ¼ cup Sophia's Seeds Formula or flax and psyllium seeds mixed in cranberry juice, followed by 2-3 cups of water; Sonia's Antioxidant Smoothie (see chapter 1) with added sprouts and 2-3 pinches of Denna's Rooibos Chai; a bowl of steamed beets and yams. Or 3-4 egg whites cooked with dill and feta cheese; and Denna's Rooibos Chai with soy or almond milk.

Mid-morning snack: Green tea; ½ cup of organic low-fat yogurt topped with ½ cup of cantaloupe or grapes, 5 almonds, and fennel seed or ginger candies.

Lunch: ¼ cup Sophia's Seeds Formula with 2 cups of water; ½ cup of hummus on a bed of arugula, watercress, or baby lettuce; tofu and mushroom soup, or vegetable and bean soup, or mixed sautéed vegetables (sprouts, chives, ginger, eggplant, baby corn, bok choy, cabbage, broccoli, carrots); 1 medium-sized Asian pear and a cup of mint or ginger tea for dessert.

Mid-afternoon snack: ½ cup of carrot juice with fresh ginger; Healthy & Wise Tea or soy chai latte; flaxseeds and sesame seeds to chew; nori seaweed sheet; 4-5 each dried cranberries and almonds.

Dinner: ¼ cup Sophia's Seeds with 2 cups of water; the baked salmon recipe, a big bunch of mixed greens, tomato, sprouts, canned or sprouted garbanzo beans, radish, onion, a slice of avocado, a pinch of sesame seeds, balsamic vinegar, and a dash of olive oil.

Before-bed snack: Peaceful & Happy Tea or chamomile tea; 1-2 dried figs or half a warmed yam wrapped in seaweed; and ½ cup of yogurt.

You can eat all the colorful vegetables, greens, and culinary herbs you want and drink as much tea as you want for any meal or snack, at any time of the day. Meditation, acupressure, and qi gong can also help your body and mind stay centered and calm during your cleansing days.

Cleansing for Food Sensitivity or Food-Related Issues

If you suspect you have a food sensitivity or allergy; or you have problems with your immune system, experience an overgrowth of candidas (otherwise known as yeast), migraines, trouble losing weight, or bad allergy attacks; or believe you might benefit from eliminating certain foods from your diet, use this more strenuous cleansing plan to solve your problem. Eat the same way as described in the cleansing plan above, but follow these additional steps:

Step 1: Begin by eliminating starchy foods and gluten-forming grains. These include wheat, oats, and barley and gluten-forming flour such as wheat, barley, oat, rye, or semolina flour. You will reintroduce them one by one to discover your food sensitivities. If you are sensitive to wheat you may be sensitive to the other gluten-forming grains. While you are eliminating the gluten-forming grains, you may eat the following gluten-free grains: brown rice, amaranth, buckwheat, quinoa, and millet. (When cutting wheat and gluten from your diet, make sure to increase other fibers like beans and bean flours; non-gluten-forming grains like buckwheat, amaranth, quinoa, millet, and kamut; fruits; vegetables; and ground flaxseeds.)

Step 2: Eliminate foods that are sugary, starchy, salty, processed, or aged or fermented (such as cheese, vinegar, and wine); and artificial foods, including diet foods and foods with artificial sweeteners, fats, and preservatives.

Step 3: List any other foods and beverages you'd like to eliminate. Begin with these:

- Foods you crave; you may find these are creating your problems.

- Processed foods and beverages; diet foods and sodas; foods and beverages with artificial sweeteners; non-organic supplements; aged or fermented foods.

- Foods that change your moods, making you feel euphoric, elated, or exhausted. The highs from caffeine and sugar feel good, but sudden mood changes caused by foods, especially when such reactions are not "normal" for those foods, can indicate food sensitivities.

- Foods that give you indigestion, cramps, excessive gas, or other uncomfortable symptoms, and foods that, according to your journal, negatively affect your mental or physical health.

- Coffee and other high-caffeine beverages, alcohol, tobacco, and any other addictive substances.

Step 4: For the next three weeks, pay attention to how you feel. List your symptoms, moods, energy levels, and other pertinent information in your food diary.

Step 5: If your major symptoms lessen or disappear, continue practicing steps 1 and 2 for two to three months.

Step 6: Reintroduce the eliminated foods to your present diet, one by one in small portions. Do not combine them with other foods you have eliminated. If you remain symptom-free, eat only that food for the next two days. For example, if you're trying to find out whether eggs cause your health symptom, eat an omelet for breakfast, an egg sandwich or hard-boiled eggs for lunch and snacks, and a frittata for dinner. This will give your body enough time to test the food.

If problems suddenly occur soon after eating the food, do not continue eating it. If no problems occur, watch for delayed responses, such as a craving, depression, mucus, bloating, or other symptoms. If there are no delayed responses, then it's okay for you to eat that food. Then check the other foods you've eliminated in the same way. Allow three to four days between testing each rein-troduced food. Keep a record of your body's responses in your food diary.

If symptoms return with the reintroduction of any food, eliminate that food from your diet. You will then know that the reintroduced food should be avoided. Read Andrew's story (earlier in this chapter) to learn how he discovered his food sensitivities using his food journal. You can also find a more extensive explana-tion of the cleansing plan in *Eating Wisely for Hormonal Balance* (Gaemi 2004).

Step 7: Medications and over-the-counter supplements can con-tribute to food allergies and sensitivities, candidas overgrowth, and other health problems. If you cannot safely stop taking medications or supplements while participating in the Eating Hormonally Cleansing Plan, be sure to ask your doctor whether taking an enzyme supplement might help your body to digest food more efficiently.

Having a homemade smoothie at any time of day is a deli-cious, easy way to make sure you get important nutrients and phytohormones without eating any of the foods you're avoiding for cleansing purposes. See chapter 1 for a recipe for a healing, all-around smoothie for any time of day or night.

Leila's Successful Cleansing

When Leila first came to Dr. Sonia's Food Wisdom Therapy clinic for help, she was consuming only 8 grams of fiber a day rather than the recommended 35 to 45 grams. She ate no essential fats and almost no fiber or phytohormonal foods. Her skin looked older than her years and she sometimes broke out in rashes all over her body. Leila was irritable, underweight, and constipated (sometimes going for two weeks without a bowel movement). She was unable to concentrate, had night sweats due to perimenopause, even though she was quite young, and frequent headaches. Over the past six years, she had had frequent yeast infections, and she had just been diagnosed with fibroid tumors (benign tumors thought to be linked to estrogen production). Because of gas and bloating, she rarely felt hungry. The foods she did eat were highly acidic, with high concentrations of starch, sugar, and hydrogenated fats.

Her symptoms suggested candidas, and a simple laboratory test proved this diagnosis correct. Sonia thought that Leila might be sensitive to gluten, so for a five-week period, Leila followed the Eating Hormonally Cleansing Plan, and eliminated wheat, barley, and other gluten-forming grains from her diet, as well as soy and sugar, and she began taking two tablespoons of psyllium husks mixed in two cups of water or unsweetened pomegranate juice every day, in addition to her Sophia's Seeds Formula.

Every day, she used her food diary to track what she ate, how she felt, her energy levels, when she experienced bloating and gas, and when bowel movements took place. After two weeks, her skin rashes and headaches disappeared and she began sleeping better. She began to have two to three bowel movements a day, and bloating and gas became rare events. Her energy level felt balanced, neither too high nor too low. She also began doing fifteen minutes of meditation or qi gong each day.

By adding new, wheat-free foods to her diet slowly (one type of grain at a time), she discovered delicious alternatives to wheat, like amaranth, millet, and quinoa. Her system thrived on these new grains, which didn't cause the hormonal imbalances that had been the cause of her previous symptoms. Amaranth cereal, sprouted buckwheat, and millet bread made with roasted garbanzo flour are now her favorite grains.

Leila's job as a magazine writer often keeps her at her desk all day, with no time for a lunch break, so the smoothies she brings to work have become her energy fix for the afternoons. Because she needs essential fatty acids, she adds an extra two tablespoons of ground flaxseeds, ground walnuts, rice bran, and fish oil to her smoothies to increase her body's absorption of nutrients. Adding essential fatty acids and tryptophan-rich foods like hummus, pumpkin seeds, yogurt, and berries helps to regulate her moods, improve her sleeping patterns, and reduce cravings. She also takes an organic multivitamin, calcium and magnesium supplements, wheat germ oil, and an organic digestive enzyme.

Leila was one of Sonia's first clients to create a unique system for herself. She decided to continue using the Eating Hormonally Cleansing Plan six days a week, eating organic low-fat yogurt, eggs, feta cheese, almond butter, or fish at least three times a week to raise her levels of amino acids. One day a week she chooses to eat the foods she misses, like meat, desserts, sodas, and creamy sauces, but she no longer craves high-fat foods. Leila's willingness to eat hormonally, experiment with foods' colors, eat mindfully, open her mind to healing techniques such as acupressure, meditation, and qi gong, and keep an accurate food diary were crucial to her successful recovery. After three months of following the cleansing plan, her fibroid tumors have shrunk in size, and she was recently able to become pregnant.

TIMES TO EAT

It's important to eat regularly through the day, and it's better to eat four to six smaller meals throughout the day than the three large meals Americans traditionally consume. Eating smaller meals throughout the day helps your body's insulin to remain steady; it also helps your body to maintain its metabolism at a constant rate.

Studies have shown that eating more frequent, smaller meals helps people to maintain a healthy weight (Ma et al. 2003) and lower cholesterol levels (Titan et al. 2001). Tracking your eating times will help you establish the best eating schedule for yourself.

The best eating schedule is not based on the times you think you're supposed to eat; rather, it's based on when you feel hungry again, after the food you ate at your previous meal has been used by your body. Judge when to eat by the signals your body sends you that it is hungry, not because it's "mealtime," you're bored or anxious, or because someone puts food in front of you.

If you eat breakfast at 8 A.M., you might be ready for a snack at 10:30, lunch by 12, a snack at 3, a lighter snack before leaving work, a satisfying but not large dinner around 6 P.M., and a light snack later in the evening. Many people feel hungry between "normal" meal times but they don't eat anything because they think it's bad to snack. They think that snacking will ruin their appetite or lead to weight gain. But ignoring normal hunger pangs can lead to insulin imbalance, food cravings, low blood sugar, fatigue, mental fogginess, and binge eating. Snacking on nutrient-dense foods like fresh or dried fruit, sprouts, leafy greens, fresh herbs and vegetables, roasted beans and seeds, or yogurt will help you maintain your energy level all day, balance your insulin, and keep unwanted weight off, and you'll find that you'll eat less at mealtimes.

If you are continually hungry, even after you've eaten, you can use your journal to figure out why. Pay attention to the meals that leave you unsatisfied and make sure you are eating hormonally, getting enough colorful, whole foods with essential fatty acids, protein, fiber, and the other elements discussed in chapter 1. Eventually, as you track your meals in the journal, you will see a pattern.

Perhaps you'll find that when you eat only simple carbohydrates at breakfast (cereal without fruit, or pastries or white toast), you get hungry faster. This may mean you need more fiber at breakfast, such as you'll find in a smoothie, an omelet, a slice or two of whole wheat bread with feta cheese or hummus, a bean dish, or some dried or fresh fruit. Record your mealtimes and snack times in your food journal and use this information to discover your natural eating schedule. Your journal will inform you about when and what to feed your body. If you keep adjusting your eating habits and continue feeling hungry most of the time, have your doctor check your blood-sugar levels to make sure you aren't developing diabetes.

FOODS TO EAT

The core concepts of the Food Wisdom Pyramid are that we should eat as many colors, textures, and tastes of whole foods as possible; eat natural foods with few or no preservatives or chemical additives; and that we should enjoy our food as much as we can. By now, you already have compiled your basic wise eating shopping list. Track what you eat at every meal, including how much you eat of each item.

For example, if you have a healthy salad at lunch, you might write that you ate the following: 1 medium bunch of spinach, lettuce, and arugula; 2 pinches of fresh parsley and dried seaweed sprinkles; about ½ cup of light tuna; a handful of sprouted organic garbanzos; one small tomato; a pinch of black pepper; a pinch of cayenne pepper; a large pinch of black sesame seeds; a small chunk of feta cheese; and a splash of virgin olive oil and balsamic vinegar.

Your journal entries don't have to include exact measurements precisely, but you do want to have some idea of how much of each food you had. Eating hormonally is not about setting rules about food portions; it's about eating a balance and variety of different kinds and colors of foods, eating enough to feel satisfied, and taking pleasure in food but not eating so much that you feel uncomfortable and bloated. Eat the amounts that satisfy you, but if you feel stuffed after a meal, record this in your journal, and at your next meal eat smaller portions to see if you feel better afterward.

Here is a colorful recipe for a tea useful for boosting energy, cleansing your system, and supporting hormone balance and immune function. The more unusual ingredients are available in natural food stores that sell medicinal herbs.

2 tbsp. each of green tea, borage flowers, and damiana leaves

4–5 each of red clover flowers and cardamom seeds

2 tbsp. rooibos leaves

I tsp. each of fennel seeds, crushed rose hips and petals, hibiscus petals, barberries, chrysanthemum petals, and black tea (optional)

Mix all the ingredients. Use 2-3 tsp. for each 1-2 cups of tea, or steep the appropriate amount in a teapot for all-day use.

Remember, eating smaller, more frequent meals is better for you than eating two or three large ones.

Tracking your food choices and quantities will help you see your eating patterns clearly and, depending on your health goals, will inform you how to change them. For example, if you have extreme energy fluctuations during the day, you'll want to try to eat fewer simple carbohydrates, starches, and sugars and more fruits, whole grains, complex carbohydrates, and protein. Or maybe you are premenopausal and wondering whether eating more phyto-hormonal foods and drinking teas like Denna's Rooibos Chai and Healthy & Wise Tea will help ease your symptoms while you pass through the stages of menopause.

By looking at the healing and wellness goals you wrote down in chapter 2, you can begin adding foods that will help you meet your goals or cutting down on foods that are not helpful. As you review your journal entries, remember to look for balance and diversity in your food choices and in the colors of your foods (see the section "Colors" later in this chapter).

YOUR MOODS AND ENERGY LEVELS

Do you tend to be energetic in the morning and then "crash" in the afternoon? This is a common problem, and your food journal will help you find out how to stabilize your energy levels throughout the day. Many of us eat colorless breakfasts high in simple carbohydrates, sugar, and caffeine, and low in whole plant foods, which can cause high insulin levels in the body and lead to diabetes, depression, and weight gain. This gives us high initial energy that's followed closely by fatigue. If you have low energy after eating lunch, discover how to maintain your energy through the afternoon by experimenting with the types and amounts of foods you eat at lunch. It may be a simple matter of eating a breakfast of complex carbohydrates, a smaller lunch, and snacking more often on colorful snacks like roasted garbanzos or lentils, flaxseeds, and fresh or dried fruit.

Record your energy level before each meal using a scale from 1 to 5, with 1 as the least amount of energy and 5 as the most. Energy means more than just whether we have a lot of energy or not very much. In traditional healing arts like qi gong and tai chi, and many healing traditions including Chinese, Persian, and Indian medicine, energy is understood to flow through all living organisms, including our bodies and the foods we eat. Eating hormonally is designed to help us balance the energies in our bodies and minds with the foods we eat and with the environment around us. This is why we encourage you to explore meditation, practices such as qi gong and yoga, and mindfulness. These practices help us balance our energies, affecting not only our mental state, but also how our immune system, hormones, digestion, and organs function.

Your moods are affected by the foods you eat and can also be affected by the times you eat those foods. If you tend to be irritable or to have trouble concentrating in the afternoons, this may be a sign of low blood sugar and may indicate you need to snack more often on energy-giving snacks like fruit, nuts, or seeds. You might also find that certain foods affect your moods, and that you should avoid or eat less of them. If you find that certain foods affect your mood severely, you may have a food sensitivity (see the "Cleansing" section earlier in this chapter). You may also need to help your body's digestive enzymes remain balanced by eating yogurt with live cultures, organic enzyme supplements, and following the Eating Hormonally Cleansing Plan several times a week.

COLOR, TIMING, AND ENERGY

Ancient healing wisdom from China, Persia, and Tibet links time of the day and food colors to particular body organs. If you have a problem with a particular organ, such as heart disease, recurrent bladder infections, or irritable bowel syndrome, find the affected organ on the following chart and make an effort to eat foods of the color listed. Be sure to eat a rainbow of colorful foods for prevention and healing, but eat more of the particular color that corresponds with your troublesome organ. Also, pay attention to the time of day that corresponds with the organ and be especially careful of not taxing that part of your body during that time of the day.

For instance, if you have heart problems, try not to tax your heart during the hours of 11 A.M. to 1 P.M., and remember to eat a lot of red-colored whole foods. If you have troubling symptoms at a certain time of day, find that time on the chart and concentrate on eating the corresponding color of food. If you have trouble waking up in the morning, for example, look at that time of day on the chart. Your intestines, lungs, or stomach may need support and you can try eating more natural white-colored foods for breakfast, such as egg whites, steamed turnips, cauliflower, jicama, hummus, yogurt, barley, amaranth, or oat cereal with soy or almond milk and flax or sesame seeds, with some berries added for color.

COLORS

Nature overflows with color. The sky, the water, and all living things on the earth abound with different changing, vibrant colors. We enjoy looking at colors, so why not enjoy putting them into our bodies as well? The colors in natural foods like fruits and veg-etables are beautiful, but they also let us know the food's health

Colorful Foods for Healing and Energy

Hour of the Day	Organ	Food Colors That Support These Organs
3-5 A.M.	Lung	White
5-7 A.M.	Large intestine	White & yellow
7-9 A.M.	Stomach	Yellow & green
9-11 A.M.	Spleen	Yellow & golden brown
11 A.M.-1 P.M.	Heart	Red
1-3 P.M.	Small intestine	Red & green
3-5 P.M.	Bladder	Black & brown
5-7 P.M.	Kidney	Black
7-9 P.M.	Pericardium (the sac around the heart)	Red
9-11 P.M.	Heart, spleen, kidney (triple organ energies)	Red & purple
11 P.M.-1 A.M.	Gallbladder	Green & yellow
1-3 A.M.	Liver	Green

benefits. For example, bright red fruits and vegetables like tomatoes, beets, and red peppers are high in lycopene, a type of antioxidant thought to fight heart disease and some cancers. The dark green color of vegetables like kale and watercress indicates high levels of calcium and folate, essential for the liver, gallbladder, and bones.

The more intense the color, the higher the concentration of the healthful phytohormones and antioxidants in the food. This is why the food journal includes a place to track the colors of your foods. Simply record the first letter of the color ("O" for orange, "R" for red, etc.) in the color column, or make a mark with a

Eating Hormonally for Color and Healing

Support For	Color	Foods
Gastrointestinal problems Stomach & spleen	Orange, yellow, gold, brown	Asian pear, citrus fruits, cantaloupe, persimmons, peaches, apricots, carrots, bananas, papayas, ginger, golden nuts and seeds, pumpkin, sweet potatoes, yams, squash, flaxseeds, brown rice, potatoes
Skin, colitis, allergies, immune system Lungs & colon	White, golden brown	Steamed root vegetables, daikon, psyllium husks, endive, pear, almonds, yogurt, bean sprouts, ginger, olive oil, flaxseeds, Peaceful & Happy Tea, Denna's Roobios Chai
PMS, fatigue, puberty Liver, gallbladder, pancreas, kidneys	Green, golden brown	Sprouts, culinary herbs and spices (especially mint & fennel seeds), leafy greens, green tea, cucumbers, okra, pumpkin seeds, seaweed, kiwi, green apples, green grapes, flaxseeds, rice, bran, Healthy & Wise Tea
Allergies, cravings, diabetes, menopause, weight loss Kidneys, pancreas	Black, orange, green	Black cherries, black sesame seeds, cardamom seeds, poppy seeds, black mushrooms, black walnuts, black dates, Denna's Roobios Chai
Mood Heart, bones	Red, pink, green, purple	Beets, red berries, pink grapefruit, red grapes, plums, prunes, raisins, cherries, pomegranates, rose petals & hips, hibiscus, red peppers, tomatoes, cayenne, red onions, seaweed

Be sure to eat a variety of colors, but include these colors for support of specific organs and systems.

colored pencil. Eating hormonally encourages you to include as many different colors in your diet as possible every day.

When shopping for groceries, make it a challenge to find as many different-colored fruits and vegetables as you can. Some people enjoy using different-colored pencils, crayons, or pens to record the colors of their foods. It makes the pages of the journal as bright and lively as your body and mind will be, and you can tell at a glance if you are getting more of one color than of another.

The previous chart gives you an idea of some foods that are particularly good for healing certain health conditions. As always, eat a rainbow of foods, and be sure to eat a variety of fiber, antioxidants, phytohormones, protein, and essential fats. Refer to the Food Wisdom Pyramid for suggested quantities.

PLEASURE

Taking pleasure and joy in your meals is extremely important. People who are overweight, who often experience digestion problems, or who have eating disorders may eat their food too quickly to taste it. Few things bring people together more than enjoying a meal together. Meals are a reason to take our minds off of work, relationship problems, or other worries. We pay attention then to our senses: the warmth of the meal; the scents from the cooking; the beautiful colors on our plates; and the different tastes and textures of the food; as well as to the laughter, joy, and energy we get from sharing meals with loved ones.

When you record your pleasure level in your food journal, think about how much you enjoyed the meal. Did you take a break for lunch, sitting outside in a park while you took a few minutes to breathe deeply and relax before really tasting your food and enjoying it, or did you eat it at your desk while working? Did you eat a frozen packaged meal for dinner as you watched TV, or did you make yourself a healthy meal, taking the time to savor the taste and smells of the fresh ingredients? Your pleasure level depends on what you consider enjoyable. Note that you needn't dine with others to enjoy your meals. Some people find that eating alone helps them to center themselves and is re-energizing. Your enjoyment is based on what is important to you, not to someone else.

When you take the time to consider whether you enjoyed your meal, you'll find that you pay more attention to your meals and may even begin planning ahead to make mealtimes more enjoyable. Make up your own rating system for your pleasure level, or try using 0 if the meal is completely unpleasurable and 10 if the meal was extremely enjoyable. Try to have one 9 or 10 meal each week, and then slowly increase the number so that most of your meals are in the 7 to 10 range.

Remember to use this same principle as you look at your other activities, and make it your goal to indulge in activities that bring you pleasure, love, and joy every day. Remember too that each of us has the power to love and heal ourselves, and in so doing, to love and heal the world.

FEELINGS OR SYMPTOMS

This section of the journal is where you will keep track of physical, emotional, or psychological symptoms you may experience, whether it's fatigue, insomnia, anxiety, depression, indigestion, acne, joint pain, or anything else. Symptoms are your body's way of telling you that something is out of balance somewhere. To find the causes of the imbalance, eating hormonally encourages you to first pay attention to the symptoms you're experiencing.

As you work with your journal, pay attention to your symptoms. Do you have hot flashes or headaches at the same time every afternoon? Pay attention to what you ate and drank for lunch, as well as to what was happening before your symptoms started. Did you quarrel with a coworker or get a stressful e-mail, or are you crashing from too much coffee in the morning? Making a change to your daily routine may help. Drink a latte made with Denna's Rooibos Chai and soy or almond milk instead of coffee or soda. Do some simple stretches or self-acupressure, take a break from work for a short meditation, or take a walk around the block in the late morning.

As you continue working with your journal, you will notice patterns to your symptoms. Then you can experiment with your foods, movement, meditation, or other daily "quiet mind" practices like qi gong, yoga, walking, dancing, gardening, or just calmly sitting, to see how your experience changes. These changes may bring more relaxation, joy, and mindfulness to your life.

GOALS FOR TOMORROW

A commitment to eating and living wisely must start with a goal. In chapter 2 you listed your long-term health and lifestyle goals, whether to lose weight, prevent PMS or menopausal symptoms, control your diabetes, have more energy, bring more joy into your life, or heal symptoms of a chronic condition. Now, using your journal pages, you can work on small goals that, when combined, will help you meet your long-term goals. For example, if you want to lose weight, your goal may be to begin with a week's cleansing and future goals may be to eat hormonally and take thirty minutes a day to do moderate exercise. If you struggle with depression, you may want to choose a goal of taking a cleansing day once a week, eating hormonally three to four times a week and spending ten to fifteen minutes a day meditating or participating in another "quiet mind" activity like yoga, qi gong, walking, or sitting quietly in a beautiful place and doing deep breathing.

Your goal for the day can be as simple as "Take ten minutes at lunch to sit in the park and savor some tea instead of eating at my desk," "Eat one of every color fruit or vegetable," or "Drink Sophia's Seeds Formula twice a week." Your goal can be the same every day. ("Cultivate a joyful attitude.") Or it can be different every day, depending on your plans for that day. ("Take ten minutes at the break in our daylong meeting to have a cup of tea and do some simple self-acupressure.") At the end of the day, take some time to reflect on whether you met your goal, and what the circumstances were. If you didn't reach that day's goal, perhaps tomorrow you can set yourself a simpler goal, or spend some time reflecting on how to reach that same goal in the future. It's important not to be too tied to your goals, but to be flexible and joyful in your attitude toward them. In chapter 5 we will discuss this in greater depth.

THE JOURNAL PAGE

The journal itself is the heart of this book. A sample filled-in page follows, and in chapter 4 you will find six weeks of blank pages to use to record the foods you eat, your moods, energy levels, and all the other aspects of wise eating and living that we've discussed. Remember, it's your journal, and you are encouraged to use it in any way that works for you. After several weeks of taking notes in your food journal, you will have much greater insight into how your body and mind work and what you need from food to feel healthy, energetic, young, and joyful.

Now, you are ready to take responsibility for your life and health by using the food journal. Before you begin, congratulate yourself for taking the first step of picking up this book.

Sample Journal Page

Date: 8/04/05	Mood & Thoughts on Waking: *Tired when I woke up, didn't want to go to work. Kept thinking about the deadline today. It's cloudy today.*

Movement	Meditation/Breathing	Cleansing
type: *qi gong, walking*	type: *Breathing, Meditation*	yes / (no)
time: *30 min, 15 min*	time: *10 min, 15 min*	

	Food eaten?	Food colors?	How do you feel?
BREAKFAST hunger level 5+ time eaten 8:15 pleasure level 5	*Bran flakes w/ raisins, dried cranberries, fresh blueberries; ½ c soy milk, ½ c almond milk; 1 slice wheat toast w/ honey; 1 c Healthy & Wise Tea.*	*Brown, red, blue, white*	*Headache, breaking out on chin, constipated. Anxious, depressed, low energy* energy level 3
SNACK hunger level 2 time eaten pleasure level	*None, waiting for lunch*		*Hungry, a little light-headed, cranky, depressed* energy level 3
LUNCH hunger level 5 time eaten 1:30 pleasure level 7	*½ chicken sandwich on sourdough baguette, sprouts & greens w/ vinaigrette dressing; chai tea; small cup of lentil soup*	*White, green, red, brown*	*Felt stuffed. Still a little headache but lunch was fun.* energy level 4
SNACK hunger level 3 time eaten 3:00 pleasure level 5	*Cantaloupe and peach, cut up, cup of Denna's Rooibos Chai*	*Orange, red*	*Headache gone. A little depressed, ready to go home.* energy level 3
DINNER hunger level 4 time eaten 7:15 pleasure level 8	*About 1 ½ cups of brown rice & broccoli, half a salmon fillet w/ sage and black pepper, cranberry juice*	*Brown, pink, black, red, green*	*I feel better, less tired and depressed. We had fun and laughed a lot.* energy level 5
SNACK hunger level 4 time eaten 9:30 pleasure level 6	*2 dried figs wrapped in seaweed, ½ cup of yogurt, cup of chamomile tea*	*brown white*	*sleepy, no headache* energy level 3

Goals for Tomorrow: *Keep eating red and purple foods for depression. Ask Katie to a movie, or on a walk for lunch.*

Your Food Journal

In chapter 4 you'll find six weeks of blank journal pages to fill out. Remember that keeping this food journal should be fun. Use it as often as you like, and if you forget to record a meal or even an entire day, don't give up. Although the journal is most useful if used every day for six weeks, patterns will emerge even if it is used less consistently. The most important thing to remember about using this journal is that, by picking it up in the first place, you've made an important step toward becoming your own healing and lifestyle coach by taking action to improve your life, your physical health, and your mental well-being. Enjoy the discoveries you'll make with this journal and keep an open mind. When you are done with the pages, keep this book in your kitchen for inspiration.

chapter 4
your food journal pages

Date:	Mood & Thoughts on Waking:

Movement	Meditation/Breathing	Cleansing
type:	type:	yes / no
time:	time:	

	Food eaten?	Food colors?	How do you feel?
BREAKFAST hunger level time eaten pleasure level			energy level
SNACK hunger level time eaten pleasure level			energy level
LUNCH hunger level time eaten pleasure level			energy level
SNACK hunger level time eaten pleasure level			energy level
DINNER hunger level time eaten pleasure level			energy level
SNACK hunger level time eaten pleasure level			energy level

Goals for Tomorrow:

Date: _____ Mood & Thoughts on Waking: _____

_____

Movement	Meditation/Breathing	Cleansing
type: _____	type: _____	yes / no
time: _____	time: _____	

	Food eaten?	Food colors?	How do you feel?
BREAKFAST hunger level time eaten pleasure level			energy level
SNACK hunger level time eaten pleasure level			energy level
LUNCH hunger level time eaten pleasure level			energy level
SNACK hunger level time eaten pleasure level			energy level
DINNER hunger level time eaten pleasure level			energy level
SNACK hunger level time eaten pleasure level			energy level

Goals for Tomorrow: _____

Date: _____ Mood & Thoughts on Waking: _____

_____

_____

Movement	Meditation/Breathing	Cleansing
type: _____	type: _____	yes / no
time: _____	time: _____	

	Food eaten?	Food colors?	How do you feel?
BREAKFAST hunger level ____ time eaten ____ pleasure level ____			energy level ____
SNACK hunger level ____ time eaten ____ pleasure level ____			energy level ____
LUNCH hunger level ____ time eaten ____ pleasure level ____			energy level ____
SNACK hunger level ____ time eaten ____ pleasure level ____			energy level ____
DINNER hunger level ____ time eaten ____ pleasure level ____			energy level ____
SNACK hunger level ____ time eaten ____ pleasure level ____			energy level ____

Goals for Tomorrow: _____

Date: _____ Mood & Thoughts on Waking: _____

_____

Movement	Meditation/Breathing	Cleansing
type: _____	type: _____	yes / no
time: _____	time: _____	

	Food eaten?	Food colors?	How do you feel?
BREAKFAST hunger level _____ time eaten _____ pleasure level _____			energy level _____
SNACK hunger level _____ time eaten _____ pleasure level _____			energy level _____
LUNCH hunger level _____ time eaten _____ pleasure level _____			energy level _____
SNACK hunger level _____ time eaten _____ pleasure level _____			energy level _____
DINNER hunger level _____ time eaten _____ pleasure level _____			energy level _____
SNACK hunger level _____ time eaten _____ pleasure level _____			energy level _____

Goals for Tomorrow: _____

Date:	Mood & Thoughts on Waking:

Movement	Meditation/Breathing	Cleansing
type:	type:	yes / no
time:	time:	

	Food eaten?	Food colors?	How do you feel?
BREAKFAST hunger level time eaten pleasure level			energy level
SNACK hunger level time eaten pleasure level			energy level
LUNCH hunger level time eaten pleasure level			energy level
SNACK hunger level time eaten pleasure level			energy level
DINNER hunger level time eaten pleasure level			energy level
SNACK hunger level time eaten pleasure level			energy level

Goals for Tomorrow:

Date: _____ Mood & Thoughts on Waking: _____

_____

Movement	Meditation/Breathing	Cleansing
type: _____	type: _____	yes / no
time: _____	time: _____	

	Food eaten?	Food colors?	How do you feel?
BREAKFAST hunger level ____ time eaten ____ pleasure level ____			energy level ____
SNACK hunger level ____ time eaten ____ pleasure level ____			energy level ____
LUNCH hunger level ____ time eaten ____ pleasure level ____			energy level ____
SNACK hunger level ____ time eaten ____ pleasure level ____			energy level ____
DINNER hunger level ____ time eaten ____ pleasure level ____			energy level ____
SNACK hunger level ____ time eaten ____ pleasure level ____			energy level ____

Goals for Tomorrow: _____

Date: _____	Mood & Thoughts on Waking: _____

Movement	Meditation/Breathing	Cleansing
type: _____	type: _____	yes / no
time: _____	time: _____	

	Food eaten?	Food colors?	How do you feel?
BREAKFAST hunger level _____ time eaten _____ pleasure level _____			energy level _____
SNACK hunger level _____ time eaten _____ pleasure level _____			energy level _____
LUNCH hunger level _____ time eaten _____ pleasure level _____			energy level _____
SNACK hunger level _____ time eaten _____ pleasure level _____			energy level _____
DINNER hunger level _____ time eaten _____ pleasure level _____			energy level _____
SNACK hunger level _____ time eaten _____ pleasure level _____			energy level _____

Goals for Tomorrow: _____

Date:	Mood & Thoughts on Waking:		

Movement	Meditation/Breathing	Cleansing
type:	type:	yes / no
time:	time:	

	Food eaten?	Food colors?	How do you feel?
BREAKFAST hunger level time eaten pleasure level			energy level
SNACK hunger level time eaten pleasure level			energy level
LUNCH hunger level time eaten pleasure level			energy level
SNACK hunger level time eaten pleasure level			energy level
DINNER hunger level time eaten pleasure level			energy level
SNACK hunger level time eaten pleasure level			energy level

Goals for Tomorrow:

Date: _____ Mood & Thoughts on Waking: _____

_____

Movement	Meditation/Breathing	Cleansing
type: _____	type: _____	yes / no
time: _____	time: _____	

	Food eaten?	Food colors?	How do you feel?
BREAKFAST hunger level ____ time eaten ____ pleasure level ____			energy level ____
SNACK hunger level ____ time eaten ____ pleasure level ____			energy level ____
LUNCH hunger level ____ time eaten ____ pleasure level ____			energy level ____
SNACK hunger level ____ time eaten ____ pleasure level ____			energy level ____
DINNER hunger level ____ time eaten ____ pleasure level ____			energy level ____
SNACK hunger level ____ time eaten ____ pleasure level ____			energy level ____

Goals for Tomorrow: _____

Date: _____ Mood & Thoughts on Waking: _____

_____

Movement	Meditation/Breathing	Cleansing
type: _____	type: _____	yes / no
time: _____	time: _____	

	Food eaten?	Food colors?	How do you feel?
BREAKFAST hunger level _____ time eaten _____ pleasure level _____			energy level _____
SNACK hunger level _____ time eaten _____ pleasure level _____			energy level _____
LUNCH hunger level _____ time eaten _____ pleasure level _____			energy level _____
SNACK hunger level _____ time eaten _____ pleasure level _____			energy level _____
DINNER hunger level _____ time eaten _____ pleasure level _____			energy level _____
SNACK hunger level _____ time eaten _____ pleasure level _____			energy level _____

Goals for Tomorrow: _____

Date:	Mood & Thoughts on Waking:

Movement	Meditation/Breathing	Cleansing
type:	type:	yes / no
time:	time:	

	Food eaten?	Food colors?	How do you feel?
BREAKFAST hunger level ___ time eaten ___ pleasure level ___			energy level ___
SNACK hunger level ___ time eaten ___ pleasure level ___			energy level ___
LUNCH hunger level ___ time eaten ___ pleasure level ___			energy level ___
SNACK hunger level ___ time eaten ___ pleasure level ___			energy level ___
DINNER hunger level ___ time eaten ___ pleasure level ___			energy level ___
SNACK hunger level ___ time eaten ___ pleasure level ___			energy level ___

Goals for Tomorrow:

Date: _____ Mood & Thoughts on Waking: _____

_____

Movement	Meditation/Breathing	Cleansing
type: _____	type: _____	yes / no
time: _____	time: _____	

	Food eaten?	Food colors?	How do you feel?
BREAKFAST hunger level _____ time eaten _____ pleasure level _____			energy level _____
SNACK hunger level _____ time eaten _____ pleasure level _____			energy level _____
LUNCH hunger level _____ time eaten _____ pleasure level _____			energy level _____
SNACK hunger level _____ time eaten _____ pleasure level _____			energy level _____
DINNER hunger level _____ time eaten _____ pleasure level _____			energy level _____
SNACK hunger level _____ time eaten _____ pleasure level _____			energy level _____

Goals for Tomorrow: _____

Date: _____ Mood & Thoughts on Waking: _____

_____

Movement	Meditation/Breathing	Cleansing
type: _____	type: _____	yes / no
time: _____	time: _____	

	Food eaten?	Food colors?	How do you feel?
BREAKFAST hunger level ____ time eaten ____ pleasure level ____			energy level ____
SNACK hunger level ____ time eaten ____ pleasure level ____			energy level ____
LUNCH hunger level ____ time eaten ____ pleasure level ____			energy level ____
SNACK hunger level ____ time eaten ____ pleasure level ____			energy level ____
DINNER hunger level ____ time eaten ____ pleasure level ____			energy level ____
SNACK hunger level ____ time eaten ____ pleasure level ____			energy level ____

Goals for Tomorrow: _____

Date:	Mood & Thoughts on Waking:			

Movement	Meditation/Breathing	Cleansing
type:	type:	yes / no
time:	time:	

	Food eaten?	Food colors?	How do you feel?
BREAKFAST hunger level time eaten pleasure level			 energy level
SNACK hunger level time eaten pleasure level			 energy level
LUNCH hunger level time eaten pleasure level			 energy level
SNACK hunger level time eaten pleasure level			 energy level
DINNER hunger level time eaten pleasure level			 energy level
SNACK hunger level time eaten pleasure level			 energy level

Goals for Tomorrow:

Date:	Mood & Thoughts on Waking:			

Movement	Meditation/Breathing	Cleansing
type:	type:	yes / no
time:	time:	

	Food eaten?	Food colors?	How do you feel?
BREAKFAST hunger level ___ time eaten ___ pleasure level ___			energy level ___
SNACK hunger level ___ time eaten ___ pleasure level ___			energy level ___
LUNCH hunger level ___ time eaten ___ pleasure level ___			energy level ___
SNACK hunger level ___ time eaten ___ pleasure level ___			energy level ___
DINNER hunger level ___ time eaten ___ pleasure level ___			energy level ___
SNACK hunger level ___ time eaten ___ pleasure level ___			energy level ___

Goals for Tomorrow:

Date: _____   Mood & Thoughts on Waking: _____

_____

Movement	Meditation/Breathing	Cleansing
type: _____	type: _____	yes / no
time: _____	time: _____	

	Food eaten?	Food colors?	How do you feel?
BREAKFAST hunger level _____ time eaten _____ pleasure level _____			energy level _____
SNACK hunger level _____ time eaten _____ pleasure level _____			energy level _____
LUNCH hunger level _____ time eaten _____ pleasure level _____			energy level _____
SNACK hunger level _____ time eaten _____ pleasure level _____			energy level _____
DINNER hunger level _____ time eaten _____ pleasure level _____			energy level _____
SNACK hunger level _____ time eaten _____ pleasure level _____			energy level _____

Goals for Tomorrow: _____

Date:	Mood & Thoughts on Waking:

Movement	Meditation/Breathing	Cleansing
type:	type:	yes / no
time:	time:	

	Food eaten?	Food colors?	How do you feel?
BREAKFAST hunger level ___ time eaten ___ pleasure level ___			energy level ___
SNACK hunger level ___ time eaten ___ pleasure level ___			energy level ___
LUNCH hunger level ___ time eaten ___ pleasure level ___			energy level ___
SNACK hunger level ___ time eaten ___ pleasure level ___			energy level ___
DINNER hunger level ___ time eaten ___ pleasure level ___			energy level ___
SNACK hunger level ___ time eaten ___ pleasure level ___			energy level ___

Goals for Tomorrow:

Date:	Mood & Thoughts on Waking:

Movement	Meditation/Breathing	Cleansing
type:	type:	yes / no
time:	time:	

	Food eaten?	Food colors?	How do you feel?
BREAKFAST hunger level time eaten pleasure level			energy level
SNACK hunger level time eaten pleasure level			energy level
LUNCH hunger level time eaten pleasure level			energy level
SNACK hunger level time eaten pleasure level			energy level
DINNER hunger level time eaten pleasure level			energy level
SNACK hunger level time eaten pleasure level			energy level

Goals for Tomorrow:

Date: _____ Mood & Thoughts on Waking: _____

_____

Movement	Meditation/Breathing	Cleansing
type: _____	type: _____	yes / no
time: _____	time: _____	

	Food eaten?	Food colors?	How do you feel?
BREAKFAST hunger level _____ time eaten _____ pleasure level _____			energy level _____
SNACK hunger level _____ time eaten _____ pleasure level _____			energy level _____
LUNCH hunger level _____ time eaten _____ pleasure level _____			energy level _____
SNACK hunger level _____ time eaten _____ pleasure level _____			energy level _____
DINNER hunger level _____ time eaten _____ pleasure level _____			energy level _____
SNACK hunger level _____ time eaten _____ pleasure level _____			energy level _____

Goals for Tomorrow: _____

Date:	Mood & Thoughts on Waking:

Movement	Meditation/Breathing	Cleansing
type:	type:	yes / no
time:	time:	

	Food eaten?	Food colors?	How do you feel?
BREAKFAST hunger level time eaten pleasure level			 energy level
SNACK hunger level time eaten pleasure level			 energy level
LUNCH hunger level time eaten pleasure level			 energy level
SNACK hunger level time eaten pleasure level			 energy level
DINNER hunger level time eaten pleasure level			 energy level
SNACK hunger level time eaten pleasure level			 energy level

Goals for Tomorrow:

Date:	Mood & Thoughts on Waking:

Movement	Meditation/Breathing	Cleansing
type:	type:	yes / no
time:	time:	

	Food eaten?	Food colors?	How do you feel?
BREAKFAST hunger level time eaten pleasure level			energy level
SNACK hunger level time eaten pleasure level			energy level
LUNCH hunger level time eaten pleasure level			energy level
SNACK hunger level time eaten pleasure level			energy level
DINNER hunger level time eaten pleasure level			energy level
SNACK hunger level time eaten pleasure level			energy level

Goals for Tomorrow:

| Date: | | Mood & Thoughts on Waking: | | |

Movement	Meditation/Breathing	Cleansing
type:	type:	yes / no
time:	time:	

	Food eaten?	Food colors?	How do you feel?
BREAKFAST hunger level time eaten pleasure level			energy level
SNACK hunger level time eaten pleasure level			energy level
LUNCH hunger level time eaten pleasure level			energy level
SNACK hunger level time eaten pleasure level			energy level
DINNER hunger level time eaten pleasure level			energy level
SNACK hunger level time eaten pleasure level			energy level

Goals for Tomorrow:

Date:	Mood & Thoughts on Waking:

Movement	Meditation/Breathing	Cleansing
type:	type:	yes / no
time:	time:	

	Food eaten?	Food colors?	How do you feel?
BREAKFAST hunger level time eaten pleasure level			energy level
SNACK hunger level time eaten pleasure level			energy level
LUNCH hunger level time eaten pleasure level			energy level
SNACK hunger level time eaten pleasure level			energy level
DINNER hunger level time eaten pleasure level			energy level
SNACK hunger level time eaten pleasure level			energy level

Goals for Tomorrow:

Date: _____ Mood & Thoughts on Waking: _____

_____

_____

Movement	Meditation/Breathing	Cleansing
type: _____	type: _____	yes / no
time: _____	time: _____	

	Food eaten?	Food colors?	How do you feel?
BREAKFAST hunger level ____ time eaten ____ pleasure level ____			energy level ____
SNACK hunger level ____ time eaten ____ pleasure level ____			energy level ____
LUNCH hunger level ____ time eaten ____ pleasure level ____			energy level ____
SNACK hunger level ____ time eaten ____ pleasure level ____			energy level ____
DINNER hunger level ____ time eaten ____ pleasure level ____			energy level ____
SNACK hunger level ____ time eaten ____ pleasure level ____			energy level ____

Goals for Tomorrow: _____

Date: _____	Mood & Thoughts on Waking: _____

_____

_____

Movement	Meditation/Breathing	Cleansing
type: _____	type: _____	yes / no
time: _____	time: _____	

	Food eaten?	Food colors?	How do you feel?
BREAKFAST hunger level ___ time eaten ___ pleasure level ___			energy level ___
SNACK hunger level ___ time eaten ___ pleasure level ___			energy level ___
LUNCH hunger level ___ time eaten ___ pleasure level ___			energy level ___
SNACK hunger level ___ time eaten ___ pleasure level ___			energy level ___
DINNER hunger level ___ time eaten ___ pleasure level ___			energy level ___
SNACK hunger level ___ time eaten ___ pleasure level ___			energy level ___

Goals for Tomorrow: _____

Date: _____ Mood & Thoughts on Waking: _____

_____

_____

Movement	Meditation/Breathing	Cleansing
type: _____	type: _____	yes / no
time: _____	time: _____	

	Food eaten?	Food colors?	How do you feel?
BREAKFAST hunger level ____ time eaten ____ pleasure level ____			energy level ____
SNACK hunger level ____ time eaten ____ pleasure level ____			energy level ____
LUNCH hunger level ____ time eaten ____ pleasure level ____			energy level ____
SNACK hunger level ____ time eaten ____ pleasure level ____			energy level ____
DINNER hunger level ____ time eaten ____ pleasure level ____			energy level ____
SNACK hunger level ____ time eaten ____ pleasure level ____			energy level ____

Goals for Tomorrow: _____

Date: _____ Mood & Thoughts on Waking: _____

_____

Movement	Meditation/Breathing	Cleansing
type: _____	type: _____	yes / no
time: _____	time: _____	

	Food eaten?	Food colors?	How do you feel?
BREAKFAST hunger level _____ time eaten _____ pleasure level _____			energy level _____
SNACK hunger level _____ time eaten _____ pleasure level _____			energy level _____
LUNCH hunger level _____ time eaten _____ pleasure level _____			energy level _____
SNACK hunger level _____ time eaten _____ pleasure level _____			energy level _____
DINNER hunger level _____ time eaten _____ pleasure level _____			energy level _____
SNACK hunger level _____ time eaten _____ pleasure level _____			energy level _____

Goals for Tomorrow: _____

Date:	Mood & Thoughts on Waking:

Movement	Meditation/Breathing	Cleansing
type:	type:	yes / no
time:	time:	

	Food eaten?	Food colors?	How do you feel?
BREAKFAST hunger level time eaten pleasure level			energy level
SNACK hunger level time eaten pleasure level			energy level
LUNCH hunger level time eaten pleasure level			energy level
SNACK hunger level time eaten pleasure level			energy level
DINNER hunger level time eaten pleasure level			energy level
SNACK hunger level time eaten pleasure level			energy level

Goals for Tomorrow:

Date:	Mood & Thoughts on Waking:

Movement	Meditation/Breathing	Cleansing
type:	type:	yes / no
time:	time:	

	Food eaten?	Food colors?	How do you feel?
BREAKFAST hunger level ____ time eaten ____ pleasure level ____			energy level ____
SNACK hunger level ____ time eaten ____ pleasure level ____			energy level ____
LUNCH hunger level ____ time eaten ____ pleasure level ____			energy level ____
SNACK hunger level ____ time eaten ____ pleasure level ____			energy level ____
DINNER hunger level ____ time eaten ____ pleasure level ____			energy level ____
SNACK hunger level ____ time eaten ____ pleasure level ____			energy level ____

Goals for Tomorrow: _____

Date: _____ Mood & Thoughts on Waking: _____

_____

Movement	Meditation/Breathing	Cleansing
type: _____	type: _____	yes / no
time: _____	time: _____	

	Food eaten?	Food colors?	How do you feel?
BREAKFAST hunger level _____ time eaten _____ pleasure level _____			energy level _____
SNACK hunger level _____ time eaten _____ pleasure level _____			energy level _____
LUNCH hunger level _____ time eaten _____ pleasure level _____			energy level _____
SNACK hunger level _____ time eaten _____ pleasure level _____			energy level _____
DINNER hunger level _____ time eaten _____ pleasure level _____			energy level _____
SNACK hunger level _____ time eaten _____ pleasure level _____			energy level _____

Goals for Tomorrow: _____

| Date: | Mood & Thoughts on Waking: |

Movement	Meditation/Breathing	Cleansing
type:	type:	yes / no
time:	time:	

	Food eaten?	Food colors?	How do you feel?
BREAKFAST hunger level time eaten pleasure level			energy level
SNACK hunger level time eaten pleasure level			energy level
LUNCH hunger level time eaten pleasure level			energy level
SNACK hunger level time eaten pleasure level			energy level
DINNER hunger level time eaten pleasure level			energy level
SNACK hunger level time eaten pleasure level			energy level

Goals for Tomorrow:

Date: _____ Mood & Thoughts on Waking: _____

_____

Movement	Meditation/Breathing	Cleansing
type: _____	type: _____	yes / no
time: _____	time: _____	

	Food eaten?	Food colors?	How do you feel?
BREAKFAST hunger level _____ time eaten pleasure level _____			energy level _____
SNACK hunger level _____ time eaten pleasure level _____			energy level _____
LUNCH hunger level _____ time eaten pleasure level _____			energy level _____
SNACK hunger level _____ time eaten pleasure level _____			energy level _____
DINNER hunger level _____ time eaten pleasure level _____			energy level _____
SNACK hunger level _____ time eaten pleasure level _____			energy level _____

Goals for Tomorrow: _____

Date:	Mood & Thoughts on Waking:

Movement	Meditation/Breathing	Cleansing
type:	type:	yes / no
time:	time:	

	Food eaten?	Food colors?	How do you feel?
BREAKFAST hunger level time eaten pleasure level			 energy level
SNACK hunger level time eaten pleasure level			 energy level
LUNCH hunger level time eaten pleasure level			 energy level
SNACK hunger level time eaten pleasure level			 energy level
DINNER hunger level time eaten pleasure level			 energy level
SNACK hunger level time eaten pleasure level			 energy level

Goals for Tomorrow:

Date: _____ Mood & Thoughts on Waking: _____

_____

Movement	Meditation/Breathing	Cleansing
type: _____	type: _____	yes / no
time: _____	time: _____	

	Food eaten?	Food colors?	How do you feel?
BREAKFAST hunger level _____ time eaten _____ pleasure level _____			energy level _____
SNACK hunger level _____ time eaten _____ pleasure level _____			energy level _____
LUNCH hunger level _____ time eaten _____ pleasure level _____			energy level _____
SNACK hunger level _____ time eaten _____ pleasure level _____			energy level _____
DINNER hunger level _____ time eaten _____ pleasure level _____			energy level _____
SNACK hunger level _____ time eaten _____ pleasure level _____			energy level _____

Goals for Tomorrow: _____

Date: _____ Mood & Thoughts on Waking: _____

_____

Movement	Meditation/Breathing	Cleansing
type: _____	type: _____	yes / no
time: _____	time: _____	

	Food eaten?	Food colors?	How do you feel?
BREAKFAST hunger level _____ time eaten _____ pleasure level _____			energy level _____
SNACK hunger level _____ time eaten _____ pleasure level _____			energy level _____
LUNCH hunger level _____ time eaten _____ pleasure level _____			energy level _____
SNACK hunger level _____ time eaten _____ pleasure level _____			energy level _____
DINNER hunger level _____ time eaten _____ pleasure level _____			energy level _____
SNACK hunger level _____ time eaten _____ pleasure level _____			energy level _____

Goals for Tomorrow: _____

Date: _____ Mood & Thoughts on Waking: _____

_____

Movement	Meditation/Breathing	Cleansing
type: _____	type: _____	yes / no
time: _____	time: _____	

	Food eaten?	Food colors?	How do you feel?
BREAKFAST hunger level ___ time eaten ___ pleasure level ___			energy level ___
SNACK hunger level ___ time eaten ___ pleasure level ___			energy level ___
LUNCH hunger level ___ time eaten ___ pleasure level ___			energy level ___
SNACK hunger level ___ time eaten ___ pleasure level ___			energy level ___
DINNER hunger level ___ time eaten ___ pleasure level ___			energy level ___
SNACK hunger level ___ time eaten ___ pleasure level ___			energy level ___

Goals for Tomorrow: _____

| Date: | | Mood & Thoughts on Waking: | | |

Movement	Meditation/Breathing	Cleansing
type:	type:	yes / no
time:	time:	

	Food eaten?	Food colors?	How do you feel?
BREAKFAST hunger level ____ time eaten ____ pleasure level ____			energy level ____
SNACK hunger level ____ time eaten ____ pleasure level ____			energy level ____
LUNCH hunger level ____ time eaten ____ pleasure level ____			energy level ____
SNACK hunger level ____ time eaten ____ pleasure level ____			energy level ____
DINNER hunger level ____ time eaten ____ pleasure level ____			energy level ____
SNACK hunger level ____ time eaten ____ pleasure level ____			energy level ____

Goals for Tomorrow:

Date: _____ Mood & Thoughts on Waking: _____

_____

Movement	Meditation/Breathing	Cleansing
type: _____	type: _____	yes / no
time: _____	time: _____	

	Food eaten?	Food colors?	How do you feel?
BREAKFAST hunger level _____ time eaten _____ pleasure level _____			energy level _____
SNACK hunger level _____ time eaten _____ pleasure level _____			energy level _____
LUNCH hunger level _____ time eaten _____ pleasure level _____			energy level _____
SNACK hunger level _____ time eaten _____ pleasure level _____			energy level _____
DINNER hunger level _____ time eaten _____ pleasure level _____			energy level _____
SNACK hunger level _____ time eaten _____ pleasure level _____			energy level _____

Goals for Tomorrow: _____

Date:	Mood & Thoughts on Waking:

Movement	Meditation/Breathing	Cleansing
type:	type:	yes / no
time:	time:	

	Food eaten?	Food colors?	How do you feel?
BREAKFAST hunger level time eaten pleasure level			energy level
SNACK hunger level time eaten pleasure level			energy level
LUNCH hunger level time eaten pleasure level			energy level
SNACK hunger level time eaten pleasure level			energy level
DINNER hunger level time eaten pleasure level			energy level
SNACK hunger level time eaten pleasure level			energy level

Goals for Tomorrow:

Date: _____	Mood & Thoughts on Waking: _____

_____

Movement	Meditation/Breathing	Cleansing
type: _____	type: _____	yes / no
time: _____	time: _____	

	Food eaten?	Food colors?	How do you feel?
BREAKFAST hunger level _____ time eaten _____ pleasure level _____			energy level _____
SNACK hunger level _____ time eaten _____ pleasure level _____			energy level _____
LUNCH hunger level _____ time eaten _____ pleasure level _____			energy level _____
SNACK hunger level _____ time eaten _____ pleasure level _____			energy level _____
DINNER hunger level _____ time eaten _____ pleasure level _____			energy level _____
SNACK hunger level _____ time eaten _____ pleasure level _____			energy level _____

Goals for Tomorrow: _____

Date:		Mood & Thoughts on Waking:		

Movement	Meditation/Breathing	Cleansing
type:	type:	yes / no
time:	time:	

	Food eaten?	Food colors?	How do you feel?
BREAKFAST hunger level time eaten pleasure level			energy level
SNACK hunger level time eaten pleasure level			energy level
LUNCH hunger level time eaten pleasure level			energy level
SNACK hunger level time eaten pleasure level			energy level
DINNER hunger level time eaten pleasure level			energy level
SNACK hunger level time eaten pleasure level			energy level

Goals for Tomorrow:

Date: _____ Mood & Thoughts on Waking: _____

_____

Movement	Meditation/Breathing	Cleansing
type: _____	type: _____	yes / no
time: _____	time: _____	

	Food eaten?	Food colors?	How do you feel?
BREAKFAST hunger level ____ time eaten ____ pleasure level ____			energy level ____
SNACK hunger level ____ time eaten ____ pleasure level ____			energy level ____
LUNCH hunger level ____ time eaten ____ pleasure level ____			energy level ____
SNACK hunger level ____ time eaten ____ pleasure level ____			energy level ____
DINNER hunger level ____ time eaten ____ pleasure level ____			energy level ____
SNACK hunger level ____ time eaten ____ pleasure level ____			energy level ____

Goals for Tomorrow: _____

chapter 5

your healing journey

A popular proverb says, "The journey of a thousand miles begins with a single step." For many of us, the thought of changing a lifetime of eating and lifestyle habits seems so challenging, we can barely manage to think about how to go about it. We say, "I'll start tomorrow." Or else we make grand plans on New Year's Day to begin a life of eating well, quitting smoking, and exercising regularly, only to give up after a few weeks and go back to our old habits. But it is possible to make these changes.

In this chapter, we'll discuss the ways that you can be your own lifestyle coach and become more responsible for your lifestyle and eating habits, based on your particular needs and priorities. By reading this journal, you've already taken the first step. Now, we'll try to help you maintain the changes you've already begun. We want to make sure you can reap the benefits of eating hormonally for the rest of your life.

Monaz's story

Monaz is a student of Sonia's who studies medicine at a prestigious university. Student life is stressful and, to save time, she used to eat her meals at the school cafeteria and she snacked on packaged snacks and coffee or diet soda. Monaz has a family history of diabetes, and weight problems, and she has spent a lot of time dieting and bingeing. Because of her chronic health problems, she has been on antibiotics several times. When she came to see Sonia for a consultation in her clinic, she was experiencing the chronic abdominal pain, gas, bloating, and lethargy of irritable bowel syndrome. Her blood-sugar level was also high.

Sonia started Monaz on the Eating Hormonally Cleansing Plan (see chapter 3) to boost her immune system, help regulate her insulin, help her body absorb nutrients more efficiently, and allow her body to rid itself naturally of toxins that had built up because of her stress and her diet high in fats, sugars, starch, and caffeine. Sonia suggested that Monaz should incude a smoothie every day with lotus seeds and fenugreek, and that she should include white-colored and bitter foods in every meal, including arugula, watercress, endive, bitter melon, apricot and grapefruit seeds, bitter almond, daikon, and Asian pear, to help heal her irritable bowel syndrome, while still getting a variety of colors in her diet.

Because of Monaz's risk of diabetes, Sonia put her on a program designed to keep her insulin levels and weight balanced. Monaz uses the Eating Hormonally Cleansing Plan once a week and plans her shopping carefully so that she eats five or six small meals each day, including a small fruit with each meal. She includes steamed cabbage, pistachios, spinach, alfalfa, turnip, coriander seeds, buckwheat, garlic, barley bread, and foods high in chromium in her diet regularly, and she sips Peaceful & Happy Tea all day as an aid for relaxation.

Monaz also began keeping a food journal, where she tracks her food using a different colored pencil for each color she eats. This way, she can see at a glance that she is eating a vibrant rainbow of foods. When she looks in her journal and sees all those bright colors on the page, it makes her feel hopeful and strong again.

When Monaz first visited Sonia, she had very little energy and got very little exercise. She drove the two miles to campus nearly every day, but once in a while, feeling guilty about her lack of exercise, she would force herself to do a strenuous workout to the point where she was exhausted or overstrained her muscles. With the energy boost she gets from her new eating habits, she now takes the thirty-minute walk back and forth from campus to her apartment at least three days a week. This not only gives her body exercise, it allows her to take a mental break from her stressful studies, slow down, and pay attention to the world around her.

Sonia also gave Monaz some suggestions for specific types of qi gong pressure points she can use on herself. These are designed to move the energy, or qi, more efficiently throughout her meridians and organs, thus relieving her lethargy and lack of energy. Sonia also suggested that Monaz should begin taking organic enzyme supplements every day in addition to greens and Healthy & Wise Tea to aid her digestion. Monaz also takes supplements of calcium, magnesium, and fresh or dried bilberry added to her tea to protect her eyes, which can be damaged by high glucose levels.

Since her discovery of eating hormonally, Monaz looks forward to bringing her new knowledge of food wisdom and healing foods to her future patients. Her classmates, seeing her weight loss, renewed energy, vibrant smile, glowing skin, and new and obvious joy in life, often ask her what her secret is. Now Monaz has healed herself with her new outlook on food, and teaches her colleagues the importance of eating joyfully and colorfully. ❧

how to begin

Earlier in this journal, you wrote down your particular healing and wellness goals. You may have written that you want to lose or gain weight, wake up refreshed, have more energy, control depression or high blood pressure, lessen the uncomfortable symptoms of PMS or menopause, or discover whether food allergies or sensitivities are causing your lethargy or abdominal bloating, or you may just want to feed your body and mind the best way you can, so you'll stay healthy and energetic, and feel fresh and young.

In these pages, we've suggested eating hormonally for all or most of your meals, getting regular physical movement, taking cleansing days, eating mindfully, drinking healing tea, making time for "quiet mind" exercises like meditation, acupressure, or solitary walks, and taking steps to heighten your enjoyment of your meals, not to mention tracking your meals every day for six weeks in this journal. What a lot of changes to make! The good news is you don't have to change your entire lifestyle overnight. ❧

discover yourself

In chapter 2, you wrote down the physical and emotional changes you are experiencing, and what you hope to achieve by using this journal. To get the most out of your new lifestyle, you'll need to know exactly what you want to happen differently in your life.

Do you want to control your depression or mood swings by paying attention to what you eat rather than taking antidepressants? Or do you want more energy so you can enjoy doing physical activities with your friends or participate in a favorite sport? Are you pregnant or planning to get pregnant and want to eat hormonally so your baby will enjoy a lifetime of good health? Are you entering menopause, or are you already past menopause, and you want to keep your bones strong, your hormones balanced, and your skin and hair hydrated and healthy? All of these goals can be achieved by mindful attention to what you put into your body as well as by adding physical and mental activities into your life designed to energize, center, or calm you. You can have more than one goal, but the important thing is to take responsibility for your own health and to know, for yourself, what you want to accomplish with this journal.

Once you've figured out your long-term goals, you can develop short-term goals for each day that you use this journal. For example, if you are trying to lose weight, you could make it a goal to get thirty to sixty minutes of fairly vigorous exercise at least four times a week. Other goals might be to do two cleansing days a week, eat a smoothie five times a week, cook one healthful recipe of foods from the low or middle part of the glycemic index (see chapter 1 for a discussion of the glycemic index) that you can use for lunches for the week, or meditate for five or ten minutes every other day followed by having a cup of your favorite tea and focusing on cultivating love and respect for your body.

EXPLORE EATING HORMONALLY

Everyone's mental and physical health and healing goals are different. However, we recommend to everyone that you base your diet on fresh foods from the Food Wisdom Pyramid that provide all the essential phytohormones, antioxidants, essential fats, fiber, protein, vitamins, and minerals that will keep your body and mind healthy. We also recommend that you balance your energy and strengthen your body with physical movement and that you spend time to calm and center your mind.

Our goal is to give you the tools you need to become your own lifestyle coach rather than depending on others to tell you how best to live your life. If you feel as if you don't know where to begin your new life of mindfulness, wise eating, and self-healing, we can point out several ways to discover the path that will fit you best.

- Sonia Gaemi's earlier book *Eating Wisely for Hormonal Balance* (2004) provides more extensive information about the Food Wisdom Pyramid and the eating hormonally program, and offers more detailed suggestions and prescriptions for healing specific health issues.

- There are many good books, CDs, DVDs, tapes, and videos that can help you. They cover topics like how to reduce stress, meditate, cope with depression, find a spiritual path, and almost any other topic you can imagine. Visit www.drsonia.com for recommendations. And visit your library or local bookstore and browse. Remember, you are the only one who knows what works for you, but others may have information that can help.

- Sign up for classes or workshops on health and wellness issues that interest you. After class, ask the instructor for ideas on ways to help yourself reach your goals.

- Join or start a self-healing group where members explore meditation, tea, qi gong, yoga, tai chi, song, dance, and other forms of self-healing.

- Consider joining an ongoing support group for people who are facing some of the same challenges you face. Groups that meet regularly can be great places to explore new ideas and develop supportive relationships to help you when you feel overwhelmed or uncertain. Look online, in your phone book, on community bulletin boards, or in your local newspaper for ongoing groups.

- Start a support group with friends for the purpose of supporting each other in self-discovery and self-coaching. You can meet regularly, have an e-mail discussion group, or find other ways to keep in touch. Check in with the progress you're making to achieve your goals, ask for ideas and input, share books, recipes, music, poems, acupressure points, health ideas, walks, adventures, movies, and videotapes. Having a strong support network can be a big help in sticking to new, healthy habits. Visit www.drsonia.com to participate in an interactive community of people interested in self-healing and eating hormonally.

- Make note of the activities you already enjoy, and figure out how to change your normal routine only slightly to add your new emotional and physical health goals. If you dislike team sports, consider ways to move your body while alone, such as qi gong, yoga, biking, walking, or swimming. If you can't stand the taste of a particular food, don't force yourself to eat it, but find another food with the same health properties and eat that instead.

- Remember, the best way to begin changing your habits is to make it just as easy to do the new habit as it was to do the old one. If you are trying to eat more healthful snacks and drink tea, be sure you have some around at all times and that they are easier to get to than the foods you are trying to eat less of. The bulk sections of natural food stores are great places to stock up on healthy snacks like almonds, walnuts, raisins, berries, other dried fruits, roasted garbanzo or soybeans, and pumpkin seeds.

- It can be both enlightening and inspiring to watch cultural programming on TV, especially when you don't have the resources or time to travel. Seeing how people from other cultures eat, think, see the world, and live their lives can give us ideas we might like to try and remind us that no matter how big the Earth is, we are all connected by our common humanity. Visit www.drsonia.com for information on how you can see Sonia's live TV show "The Art of Self Healing with Dr. Sonia." ❧

take it one step at a time

Start changing your life for the better by taking it one step at a time, making one small change until it becomes a habit, then making another change, and so on. People who try to change all of their habits at once are not usually successful. Then they blame themselves for their supposed lack of willpower when, in fact, they tried to do too much too fast. None of the emotional or physical health challenges you are dealing with developed overnight, and they won't be healed overnight. Remember, each step you take, no matter how small it seems, gets you closer to where you want to be, and each small thing you do for yourself can be a source of great joy.

It's important to meet the goals you set for yourself, but it's equally important to live in the present rather than waiting for your life to be different—for your body to be thinner, or your hot flashes to subside, or your depression to disappear—before you begin to love yourself. Although none of us will ever be perfectly fit, thin, healthy, or emotionally consistent, it's enough that we're growing and learning each day, and working with this book is an important step in taking responsibility for your own health and well-being.

This journal is the perfect tool for you to begin changing your habits slowly. Start by choosing one thing you want to do: say, eating hormonally from the Food Wisdom Pyramid for most of your meals. Plan your week around this one goal. You may want to plan your meals for the next several days to make it easy to meet your goals. For example, instead of buying a packaged sandwich and a soda every day at lunchtime, try making a homemade sandwich of avocado, sun-dried tomato, greens, and sliced red onion on whole wheat sprouted-grain bread and bringing it to work. Be sure to always have a container of tea with you, in your purse, bag, car, or desk drawer, so you can enjoy a tea break at any time. Make sure that the recipes you make follow the principles outlined here, calling for whole fruits, greens, vegetables, grains, essential fats, colorful foods, and limited amounts of oils, hydrogenated fats, sugar, and salt. The following recipe for Green Garbanzo Dill Pilaf will help you start on your way to eating hormonally:

Green Garbanzo Dill Pilaf

This therapeutic garbanzo dish is exotic, aromatic, and flavorful. Garbanzo beans are a wonderful source of antioxidants, phytohormones, protein, folic acid, and calcium. Look for sprouted garbanzos at the store, or make your own (see chapter 1). Serves 2 to 4.

2 cups long-grain, basmati, or brown rice

1 large red onion, chopped

2-3 cloves garlic, minced

2 tbsp. virgin olive oil

2 tsp. each of turmeric and cumin seeds

1 cup garbanzo beans (sprouted, canned, or home-cooked)

2 cups fresh dill, chopped, or ½ cup dried dill

1-2 tsp. pepper

Salt to taste

Pinch of saffron (optional)

Rinse the rice and soak in 5 cups of slightly salted water for 1 hour or longer. Preheat oven to 375°F. In a small pot, sauté the onion and garlic in the oil for about 5 minutes. Add the turmeric, cumin, garbanzos, and 2 cups of water, and cook for 5 minutes.

Add the remaining ingredients including the rice and its soaking water, and mix well. Place in a 3-quart glass baking dish, cover, and bake 30 to 45 minutes. Serve with scrambled eggs or a tomato omelet, fish, lamb chops, chicken or turkey breast, sautéed tofu, fresh herbs, or a green salad. Chutney, salsa, or yogurt make nice accompaniments.

If you aren't fond of garbanzos, substitute frozen green soybeans, lima beans, snow peas, or black-eyed peas.

Tip: *You can prepare this meal in your rice cooker by adding all the ingredients at once.*

Shop during the weekend for all the ingredients, doubling the recipe if you wish. As you cook, enjoy the colors and smells of the food, and the feeling of doing something good for yourself. When the pilaf is done, you will have enough to eat for the entire week, or to freeze for the following week, and you will have taken a major step in reaching your first week's goal.

Give Yourself Time to Adjust to New Habits

It takes time to get used to new habits. At first, you may miss your old habits and wonder why you changed. Friends and family may wonder, too, and may even try to make you go back to your old habits because they're more comfortable with those. When you're stressed or feeling down, it can be especially hard to stick to new habits. But don't give up. Take a deep breath, exhale deeply, and congratulate yourself for working with this book and for committing yourself to a new and healthy life.

As you explore ways of eating hormonally that will promote mental and physical healing, try not to change too much, too fast. Start slowly by picking one habit you want to change for a week. For example, you may want to start eating a healthy salad every day at lunch. Once this becomes a habit, you can change something else, such as deciding to eat a smoothie every day for breakfast or as a snack, as well as your healthy salad. Once this becomes a habit, perhaps you can sign up for a yoga, qi gong, or tai chi class one day a week. It's important to always give yourself plenty of time to adjust to your new habit before trying to change something else.

For example, if you want to balance your mood swings, you might make your first week's goal to buy some of the colored foods previously discussed that emphasize the colors red, pink, and purple. (See the chart Eating Hormonally for Color and Health in chapter 3.) Then plan and cook one recipe. In the second week, you may want to take an energy healing class such as Reiki or Breema, or a qi gong class. Or you may want to buy an instructional video or DVD and practice what you learn once or twice a week at home. In the third week you could choose to meditate every other day for five minutes a day. These incremental changes mean that by the fourth week, you'll have moved forward in each of the areas you wanted to explore.

Then, instead of signing up for another class or increasing your meditation time, keep to this schedule for several weeks, until these new habits become part of your normal routine. These may seem like small changes, but once you get into the habit of doing them every week, you'll notice that you'll feel more energized and positive, and meeting these goals each week will give you a sense of accomplishment. Visit www.drsonia.com for more support and ideas.

Once your qi gong practice, your five-minutes-every-other-day meditation, and your tasty new eating habits are part of your daily routine, then you can begin extending your meditation time. Again, start slowly, adding five minutes more to each meditation session, or an additional ten-minute session each week. Then, perhaps you'll want to practice longer qi gong sessions or take a second class. In this way, you won't feel overwhelmed by all the new activities you have to do.

Your new routine can fit into your lifestyle. Once you've established a new routine that works for you, stay with it. Good health is not a sports competition, and you don't have to deny yourself all of your favorite foods, practice a physical discipline every day, or meditate an hour a day to get good health benefits. Your new routine should fit into your life—your work, social life, family, hobbies, and other events that are important to you—not vice versa. If you know that on Tuesdays you work, take an art class, and meet your best friend for dinner, you also know that you won't have the time to do a forty-minute yoga workout or cook a recipe to eat for the rest of the week. Save the yoga and cooking for a day when you have more unscheduled time, and enjoy your workday, your art class, and your friend.

Walking meditations: You can also combine activities to meet multiple goals. For example, what if you want to walk thirty minutes a day, and meditate five to ten minutes a day, but you have trouble finding the time to do both of these things? If you take walks as part of your regular routine (for example, you walk to work or to the supermarket, or you walk your dog every evening), rather than trying to carve out more time from your busy schedule, you can do a walking meditation at the same time.

This ancient practice, still in use today, asks you to focus on your breath and give gentle attention to your body while you walk. As you take each step, be mindful of each movement your body makes. Concentrate on each breath, and when you experience a thought that wants your attention, gently let it go without dwelling on it or trying to change it. When you do a walking meditation, it provides the physical exercise of walking combined with the mental tranquillity and health benefits of meditation.

HOW TO COMMIT TO YOUR NEW HEALING LIFESTYLE

You've already made a commitment to staying strong, energetic, and healthy by reading this book. But even though we've tried to focus on the joy and creativity of eating hormonally, habits are hard to change. Each day, especially at the beginning of a new lifestyle, you will have to remind yourself to eat hormonally, to take time out for meditation, breathing, or movement, and to write in your journal while sipping healing tea. Since you're also learning new things—about what to eat, how and where to shop, how to take time out to calm and energize your mind, how to cook new recipes, and how to plan for the week—you may sometimes feel overwhelmed and think it would just be easier to go back to your old patterns. But the longer you live a life of eating hormonally, the easier it will become. Here are some ways to help yourself stay on track.

Reward Yourself Often

If you were trying to encourage a friend, or child, or even a pet, to change a habit, you'd use the reward system, so why not use it for yourself? When you meet a goal, reward yourself with something you enjoy. A weekly massage, sauna, or hot tub soak can be a great way to end the week. Or treat yourself to a cup of your favorite herb tea or chai latte in a pleasant café where you can write in your journal without being distracted. Or have a special tea ceremony for yourself, opening all of your senses to the warmth, aroma, and taste of your favorite tea recipe. Visit a part of town you've always wanted to explore, like a beautiful meditation garden. Or call or write a friend who lives far away.

Your reward doesn't have to be expensive, but it should be something out of the ordinary, something that brings you pleasure. A new book or CD, a new color of nail polish, a relaxing walk in a beautiful place, a new type of healthful dessert or tea can all be rewards you give yourself for meeting your goals.

Plan Your Time

In a society where fast food and junk food are often easier to come by than whole fruits and vegetables, the hardest part about eating hormonally can be making sure that we always have healthful foods within reach. Similarly, it's easy to plan to walk in the park during your lunch hour but then be derailed by a work project or by an invitation from a coworker to eat lunch together at a nearby fast-food restaurant. That's why planning is so important. The solution is to write down your specific plans in the same place you schedule the rest of your life, whether you use a desk calendar, handheld electronic device, pocket notebook, or your computer.

If your goal is to eat hormonally and take two cleansing days this week, schedule a time when you will do the shopping, and then schedule the days you will use for cleansing. Don't schedule a cleansing day the same day you're having dinner guests or a day you plan to go to a party. Plan your cleansing days for the times you'll have more control over the foods you'll have around. Becoming a "new you" won't happen overnight, but you'll be able to feel a difference in yourself in the first week, when you've enjoyed the colorful, flavorful, fulfilling meals that mean you are eating hormonally.

The most efficient and also the easiest way to plan for your health goals is to use the same planning tool you use for work and your social life. If you keep your healing goals separate from the rest of your life, you may be telling yourself that these goals aren't as important as the others. You'll be more likely to forget that you planned to buy groceries at the local farmer's market that day or that this is the day you've set aside twenty minutes to do some acupressure and breathing exercises after work. List your plans for the day in your regular desk calendar, handheld device, or planner, and you'll see those plans several times a day and you'll be more likely to integrate your new habits into your life.

Planning also helps you when you need encouragement. Having a visual record of your progress can help you stick to your new habits. You can look at your desk calendar and see a record of all the days you walked, took tea breaks, ate healthfully, or meditated, and you can remind yourself that you have made progress.

Build a Support Network

One of the most effective ways to begin coaching yourself to adopt a new lifestyle is to have a strong support network. People with strong interpersonal ties such as family, friends, or a supportive group heal faster from disease, lose more weight when dieting and keep it off longer, and suffer less from anxiety and depression. Food just naturally lends itself to community: sharing food in a group is the oldest human tradition. Here are some ideas for building a strong support network:

- Start a cooking club where you meet regularly to prepare food and dine together. Pick a cuisine, a particular color, or a specific food item to concentrate on for each get-together, making sure the final meal includes a variety of different colors and foods. Start an "Eating Hormonally Group" with your friends where each person tracks her food in her journal and you trade recipes, ideas, and encouragement through e-mail, phone calls, or regular get-togethers. When one or all of you meets an important goal, have a party serving foods and tea based on the ideas and recipes in this book.

- Get your family involved. Kids love to learn new things. Make shopping for healthful new foods an adventure and cook together with your kids and family members on a regular basis. Rather than viewing your new eating and lifestyle habits as restrictive, make them a new fun activity. Take family walks or bike rides after dinner, and plan family hiking trips for vacations. Hold gatherings for family and friends when you taste different healing teas. Even young kids can enjoy tea, qi gong, yoga, and walking meditation, and get the same benefits as adults.

- Pay attention to how your body feels. If your body feels stiff, move it in ways that you enjoy—dance, swim, walk, jog, do yoga, do qi gong, hike, bicycle, whatever you feel like doing. If you're cold, eat something warm and soothing or drink your favorite warming, healing tea. If you're hot, eat something cool, such as watermelon slices and a cool tea. You don't need other people to tell you what to do—you can heal yourself just by opening up to the bounty of the world.

- Bring whole foods made from organic fruits, vegetables, grains, and legumes to parties and office potlucks, and occasionally to the office, group meetings, or to share "just because." You won't be tempted to snack on donuts or junk food, and sharing food together always brings people closer.

- Attend your local farmer's market events or any festivals held in your community with the theme of self-healing and food.

Learn from Experience

There will be times when you won't meet your daily goals. You'll feel tired or have a sugar craving and will have a soda or cookies, or you'll be in a hurry and will skip breakfast, or you'll attend a friend's party and eat pepperoni pizza when your goal for the day was to eat hormonally. You might feel too exhausted to go on your nightly walk after work, or there will be an emergency you must deal with and you won't be able to meditate that morning. Sometimes life has other plans for us, and these are all okay.

Many people trying to change their habits feel guilty when they "slip up," and they go back to their old way of doing things. But guilt is not helpful, and an essential part of eating hormonally is cultivating enjoyment in your life and respect for yourself. This means that, sometimes, your body won't want that lunchtime bike ride but would rather lie down under a shady tree in the park. As long as you remain mindful of what you are trying to accomplish with your daily goals, when your goal for the day doesn't work out the way you wanted it to, be kind and loving to yourself. That day, think of something else you can feel good about, and reward yourself for it. Be open to all of life's possibilities, and love yourself as you are.

It can, however, be useful to think about what contributed to your missed goal. If your eating habits are sliding back to your old ways of eating mainly processed foods high in sugar and fats, consider what is causing you go return to those comfort foods instead of eating hormonally.

Write in your journal, meditate, or talk to a supportive friend about what is going on for you just before you make the decision to open a TV dinner or a bag of potato chips. Is it that you are tired and cooking a healthful meal will take too long? Are you frustrated because you feel deprived of some of your favorite foods? Are you stressed out with low blood sugar because you haven't eaten enough that day and just want to ease the hunger pangs no matter what? Are you being pressured by your family or living companion to resume eating the same old way?

By exploring these issues, you can come up with a plan for the future when you will feel the same way. Have healthy low- and medium-glycemic snacks on hand all the time, such as raw vegetables and hummus, yogurt, tahini, walnuts, flaxseeds, pumpkin seeds, and fresh and dried fruit. Nibble on some roasted garbanzos or dried berries before you decide what to eat for dinner. Have a talk with your partner and ask for support for your new eating habits, promising to go out for something "decadent" once a week. Reward yourself with something you love in celebration of your transformation, so you won't feel deprived. Double your recipes and freeze some wholesome meals for those times you are too tired to cook. That way you can warm them up quickly and have a ready-made, healthy dinner. Or, just eat a small portion of the food you want, so you can have the pleasure of the food without feeling as though you've somehow "failed" in your effort to eat hormonally.

When you miss your goals, there's no need to feel guilty or tell yourself you have no willpower. Make friends of your habits—both old and new—instead of enemies. Changing habits can be hard work, and instead of feeling guilty about the times you don't meet your goals, think about all the times you do meet them, and how good that it feels. You can also consider adjusting your goals. Perhaps you want to lose weight and you had the goal of eating hormonally for all your meals yesterday. But a friend had a party last night, and you ended up eating the snacks and food provided at the party. You enjoyed them, but now you feel guilty because you didn't meet your goal of eating hormonally for all your meals that day.

In the future, when you know you'll be socializing on a particular night, make your goal to have a great time at the party and meet at least one new person, and save your eating hormonally goals for the days you know you'll have more control over your environment. Another possibility would be to bring a delicious dish made from organic vegetables and grains, and share it with the other party guests. Remember, your healing goals should fit with your lifestyle, not vice versa.

A Note on Cravings

Cravings can often indicate a hormonal imbalance, imbalance in the acidity or alkalinity of the body, food sensitivity, or allergy. Sometimes the foods you crave are the problem. If you crave specific foods frequently, consider tracking these cravings in your food journal. After two weeks of tracking, follow the eating hormonally cleansing plan outlined in chapter 3, temporarily eliminating the foods you crave from your diet. Denna's Roobios Chai (see recipe in chapter 2) can be especially helpful for cravings. Pay close attention to your cravings, as well as to your energy levels and other emotional and physical changes, as you eliminate foods and slowly reintroduce them later, one by one.

If cravings or other symptoms recur after reintroducing a food, you are probably allergic or sensitive to that food and should avoid it. You also may need to focus on building up the good bacteria in your digestive system, which can be helped by eating hormonally, especially organic yogurt with active cultures, sprouts, greens, berries, flaxseeds, smoothies, Denna's Rooibos Chai, and by taking organic enzyme supplements.

Cravings may also indicate a candidas infection, which also can be helped by using the cleansing plan to eliminate and then reintroduce certain foods. If you have frequent cravings, refer to *Eating Wisely for Hormonal Balance* (Gaemi 2004), or consider consulting a registered dietitian or other health professional. If you crave certain foods during stressful times, you may need to work on your stress-management skills. Meditation, journal writing, supportive friends, and even a professional therapist can help you learn to manage stress better.

Cultivate Self-Acceptance

Many of us often think that we'd be happier or more successful if we were different. We're surrounded by advertising telling us that we should be thinner, have whiter teeth, be more outgoing, have better skin, better hair, or better jobs. Bookstores are filled with diet books advocating the newest fad diets, and many of us want to believe that, even though the last fad diet didn't work, this one will. We know that these promises are false, but still, in the back of our mind, we want to believe that, this time, the miracle cure will work.

Good health, balanced energy, strong bones, and hormonal balance are all goals we should strive for, and these are the goals the eating hormonally plan is designed to support. But, remember, none of us will ever enjoy perfect health or a complete end to pain, aging, or injury. The eating hormonally program is designed to help you discover ways to coach yourself toward a balanced and integrated body and mind, helping you to heal yourself and stay strong, alert, and healthy.

The key to living and aging gracefully is to give your body and mind the energy they need to stay healthy and vibrant and to keep a positive outlook on your life, accepting that things are never perfect, and learning to accept and learn from the imperfections, challenges, suffering, and struggles that life puts in your path. The guidelines in this book have been offered to help you have the energy to heal yourself and live a more enjoyable and more passionate life, but the joy and passion must come from inside yourself.

Spirituality

Spirituality is an important part of human experience; it can bridge the divide between mind and body and help us find a centered, tranquil space within ourselves that we can call on when we are stressed, anxious, ill, or must cope with difficult experiences. All of the ideas discussed in this book can be used in spiritual practice. Food, tea, qi gong, yoga, meditation, acupressure, opening the senses, self-healing, and self-discovery can all be important parts of any spiritual practice, no matter what religion or discipline you embrace.

Make room for spirituality and spiritual exploration in your life by joining a religious community, taking classes, participating in volunteer work, or reading books on spiritual topics that interest you.

Good Luck on Your Journey of Self-Healing and Self-Coaching

Congratulations on taking the first step toward healing your body, mind, and spirit by reading and writing in this journal. Now, go out and enjoy your life, share healing food and tea with good friends or eat a lovingly prepared meal and drink healing tea made by you for yourself. Walk, run, dance, move, meditate, breathe deeply, and laugh often.

The eating hormonally program was developed by Sonia Gaemi, who has spent thirty years researching food and nutrition and gathering wisdom from the stories and traditions of thousands of women all across the globe. In Western cultures, we are finally rediscovering the truth behind the old adage "you are what you eat." By eating colorful whole organic fruits, vegetables, greens, grains, legumes, yogurt, spices, seeds, nuts, fish, and eggs; by drinking healing tea and water; and by moving our bodies in mindful ways; we honor our senses and we influence how we feel mentally and physically.

We also influence how we age, and how we cope with the hormonal fluctuations that can manifest as weight gain, hot flashes, diabetes, PMS, high blood pressure, depression, and other challenges. Using this journal will help you understand how the energies in your body and mind react to what you put into them, and it will help you to become your own lifestyle coach, designing a life that supports you, keeps you feeling energetic and strong, and feeds your spirit.

Seven hundred and fifty years ago, the mystic and philosopher Rumi said "Happiness is a state of mind and love is the healer of all ills." We wish you the best of luck on the journey, and, remember, healing yourself is the first step toward healing the world.

references

Albertazzi P., F. Pansini, M. Bottazzi, G. Bonaccorsi, D. DeAloysio, and M. S. Morton. 1998. Dietary soy supplementation and phytoestrogen levels. *Obstetrics and Gynecology* 94(2):229-231.

Anderson, J. W. 1990. Sorting out fiber. *Saturday Evening Post* (March), http://www.findarticles.com/p/articles/mi_m1189/is_ n2_v262/ai_ 8810645

Andersen-Parrado, P. 1996. A diet rich in omega-3 fatty acids and niacinamide may help arthritis. *Better Nutrition* (October), www.findarticles.com/p/articles/mi_m0FKA/is_n10_v58/ai_ 18746176

Bernardi, L., G. Spadacini, J. Bellwon, R. Hajric, H. Roskamm, and A. W. Frey. 1998. Effect of breathing rate on oxygen saturation and exercise performance in chronic heart failure. *Lancet* 351 (9112):1308-1311.

Carlson, L. E., M. Speca, K. D. Patel, and E. Goodey. 2004. Mindful-ness-based stress reduction in relation to quality of life, mood, symptoms of stress and levels of cortisol, dehydroepiandrosterone sulfate (DHEAS) and melatonin in breast and prostate cancer out-patients. *Psychoneuroendocrinology* 29(4):448-474.

Davidson R. J., J. Kabat-Zinn, J. Schumacher, M. Rosenkranz, D. Mul-ler, S. F. Santorelli, et al. 2003. Alterations in brain and immune function produced by mindfulness meditation. *Psychosomatic Medicine* 65(4):564-570.

Dufresne C. J., and E. R. Farnworth. 2001. A review of latest research findings on the health promotion properties of tea. *Journal of Nutritional Biochemistry* 12(7):404-421.

Egan, M. E., M. Pearson, S. A. Weiner, V. Rajendran, D. Rubin, J. Glockner-Pagel, et al. 2004. Curcumin, a major constituent of turmeric, corrects cystic fibrosis defects. *Science* 304(5670):600-602.

Environmental Protection Agency. 2004. *What You Need to Know about Mercury in Fish and Shellfish.* 2004. Issued jointly by the Environmental Protection Agency and the Food and Drug Administration. http://www.epa.gov/waterscience/fishadvice/advice.html

The EURODIAB substudy 2 study group. 1999. Vitamin D supplement in early childhood and risk of Type 1 (insulin-dependent) diabetes mellitus. *Diabetalogica* 42(1):51-54.

Feskanich, D., W. C. Willett, M. J. Stampfer, and G. A. Colditz. 1996. Protein consumption and bone fractures in women. *American Journal of Epidemiology* 143:472-479.

Foster-Powell, K., S. H. Holt, and J. C. Brand-Miller. 2002. International table of glycemic index and glycemic load values. *American Journal of Clinical Nutrition* 76:5-56.

Ghaemi-Hashemi, S. A., J. A. Clarke, and S. Margen. 1998. The benefits of the Middle-Eastern food model on women's hormonal balance. *Journal of the American Dietetic Association* 98(9):A25.

Gaemi, Sonia. 2004. *Eating Wisely for Hormonal Balance.* Oakland, Calif: New Harbinger Publications.

————. 1990. *A World of Choices.* Livermore, Calif.: NutraEra.

Garland, C. F. 2003. More on preventing skin cancer: Sun avoidance will increase incidence of cancers overall. *British Medical Journal* 327: 1228.

Hayes C. E., M. T. Cantorna, and H. F. DeLuca. 1997. Vitamin D and multiple sclerosis. *Proceedings of the Society for Experimental Biology and Medicine.* 216(1):21-27.

Heaney, R. P. 1993. Nutritional factors in osteoporosis. *Annual Review of Nutrition* 13:287-316.

Hess A. F., and L. J. Unger. 1921. The cure of infantile rickets by sunlight. *Journal of the American Medical Association* 77(1):39.

Idoori, W. H., E. L. Giovannucci, H. R. Rockett, L. Sampson, E. B. Rimm, and W. C. Willett. 1998. A prospective study of dietary fiber types and symptomatic diverticular disease in men. *Journal of Nutrition* 128:714-719.

Jarvill-Taylor, K. J., R. A. Anderson, and D. J. Graves. 2001. A hydroxychalcone derived from cinnamon functions as a mimetic for insulin in 3T3-L1 adipocytes. *Journal of the American College of Nutrition* 20(4):327-336.

John, E. M., G. G. Schwartz, D. M. Dreon, and J. Koo. 1999. Vitamin D and breast cancer risk. The NHANES I epidemiological follow-up study, 1971-1975 to 1992. *Cancer Epidemiology, Biomarkers & Prevention* 8:399-406.

Johnson, J. R. 1935. The effect of carbon arc radiation on blood pressure and cardiac output. *American Journal of Physiology* 114:594-602.

Liu, S., W. C. Willett, M. J. Stampfer, F. B. Hu, M. Franz, L. Sampson, et al. 2000. A prospective study of dietary glycemic load, carbohydrate intake, and risk of coronary heart disease in US women. *American Journal of Clinical Nutrition* 71:1455-1461

Logan, A. C. 2003. Neurobehavioral aspects of omega-3 fatty acids: possible mechanisms and therapeutic value in major depression. *Alternative Medical Review* 8(4):410-425.

Ma, Y., E. R. Bertone, E. J. Stanek, III, G. W. Reed, J. R. Hebert, N. L. Cohen, et al. 2003. Association between eating patterns and obesity in a free-living U.S. adult population. *American Journal of Epidemiology* 158:85-92

MacLean, C. R., K. G. Walton, S. R. Wenneberg, D. K. Levitsky, J. P. Mandarino, R. Waziri, et al. 1997. Effects of the Transcendental Meditation program on adaptive mechanisms: Changes in hormone levels and responses to stress after four months of practice *Psychoneuroendocrinology* 22(4):277-295.

Maier, S. F., and M. Laudenslager. 1985. Stress and health: Exploring the links. *Psychology Today* (August) 19(8):44-49.

Pate, R. R., M. Pratt, S. N. Blair, W. L. Haskell, C. A. Macera, C. Bouchard, et al. 1995. Physical activity and public health: A recommendation from the Centers for Disease Control and Prevention and the American College of Sports Medicine. *Journal of the American Medical Association* 273(5):402-407.

Pelikanova, T., M. Kohout, J. Valek, J. Base, and L. Kazodva. 1989. Insulin secretion and insulin action are related to the serum phospholipid fatty acid pattern in healthy men. *Metabolic Clinical Experiments* 38:188-192.

Pennebaker, J. W. 1997. *Opening up: The Healing Power of Expressing Emotions.* New York: Guilford Press.

_____ 2003. *Writing to Heal: A Guided Journal for Recovering from Trauma & Emotional Upheaval*. Oakland, Calif.: New Harbinger Publications.

Pereira, M. A., E. O'Reilly, K. Augustsson, G. E. Fraser, U. Goldbourt, B. L. Heitmann, et al. 2004. Dietary fiber and risk of coronary heart disease: A pooled analysis of cohort studies. *Archives of Internal Medicine* 164:370-376.

Raub, J. A. 2002. Psychophysiologic effects of Hatha Yoga on musculoskeletal and cardiopulmonary function: A literature review. *The Journal of Alternative and Complementary Medicine* 8(6):797-812.

Riggs, B. L., and L. J. Melton. 1992. The prevention and treatment of osteoporosis. *New England Journal of Medicine* 327:620-627.

Sancier, K. M. 1999. Therapeutic benefits of qi gong exercises in combination with drugs. *Journal of Alternative and Complementary Medicine* 5:383-389.

Satoskar, R. R., S. J. Shah, and S. G. Shenoy. 1986. Evaluation of anti-inflammatory property of curcumin (diferuloyl methane) in patients with postoperative inflammation. *International Journal of Clinical Pharmacology, Therapy, and Toxicology* 24:651–654.

Serraino, M., and L. U. Thompson. 1992. Flaxseed supplementation and early markers of colon carcinogenesis. In *Cancer Letters* 63:159-165.

Servan-Schreiber, D. 2004. Run for your life. *Psychotherapy Networker* 47-67.

Sevrens, J. 2000. Scientists are rethinking soy's benefits. *San Jose Mercury News*, May 2.

Sherman, P. W., and J. Billings. 1998. Antimicrobial functions of spice use: Why some like it hot. *Quarterly Review of Biology* 73(1):3-49.

Siddiqui, M. Y., and M. Siddiqui. 1976. Hypolipidemic principles of *Cicer arietinum*: Biochanin-A and formononetin. *Lipids* 1:243-246.

Simopoulos, A. 1988. *Nutrition Today* March/April:12-19.

Slentz, C. A., B. D. Duscha, J. L. Johnson, K. Ketchum, L. B. Aiken, G. P. Samsa, et al. 2004. Effects of the amount of exercise on body weight, body composition, and measures of central obesity. STRRIDE—A randomized controlled study. *Archives of Internal Medicine* 164:31-39.

Spicer, D., D. Shoupe, and M. Pike. 1991. Gonadotropin-releasing hormone agonist plus add-back sex steroids to reduce risk of breast cancer. *Journal of the National Cancer Institute* 83:1763.

Titan, S., S. Bingham, A. Welsh, R. Luben, S. Oakes, N. Day, et al. 2001. Frequency of eating and concentrations of serum cholesterol in the Norfolk population of the European prospective investigation into cancer (EPIC-Norfolk): Cross-sectional study. *British Medical Journal* (December) 323:1286.

Wallace, R. K., J. Silver, P. J. Mills, M. C. Dillbeck, and D. E. Wagoner. 1983. Systolic blood pressure and long-term practice of the Transcendental Meditation and TM-Sidhi program: Effects of TM on systolic blood pressure *Psychosomatic Medicine* 45:41-46.

Wang, C., J. P. Collet, and J. Lau. 2004. The effect of Tai Chi on health outcomes in patients with chronic conditions: A systematic review. *Archives of Internal Medicine* 164:493-501.

Wrone, E. M., M. R. Camethon, L. Palaniappan, and S. P. Fortmann. 2003. Association of dietary protein intake and microalbuminuria in healthy adults: Third National Health and Nutrition Examination Survey. *American Journal of Kidney Disorders* 41:580-587.

Sonia Gaemi, Ed.D., RD, is a registered dietician who holds a doctorate in international education. She runs a nutritional consulting practice in Berkeley, CA. An internationally known expert on multicultural food practices for self-healing, she has traveled and researched extensively. She organizes and attends conferences on food and self-healing, and articles by and about her have appeared in the *San Francisco Chronicle,* the *Oakland Tribune, American Fitness Magazine, Health Medicine Forum,* and the American Dietetic Association's magazine *Courier.* She maintains a Web site at www.drsonia.com.

Melissa Kirk is an editor and writer based in the Bay Area.

Some Other
New Harbinger Titles

The Well-Ordered Office, Item 3856 $13.95

Talk to Me, Item 3317 $12.95

Romantic Intelligence, Item 3309 $15.95

Transformational Divorce, Item 3414 $13.95

The Rape Recovery Handbook, Item 3376 $15.95

Eating Mindfully, Item 3503 $13.95

Sex Talk, Item 2868 $12.95

Everyday Adventures for the Soul, Item 2981 $11.95

A Woman's Addiction Workbook, Item 2973 $18.95

The Daughter-In-Law's Survival Guide, Item 2817 $12.95

PMDD, Item 2833 $13.95

The Vulvodynia Survival Guide, Item 2914 $15.95

Love Tune-Ups, Item 2744 $10.95

The Deepest Blue, Item 2531 $13.95

The 50 Best Ways to Simplify Your Life, Item 2558 $11.95

Brave New You, Item 2590 $13.95

Loving Your Teenage Daughter, Item 2620 $14.95

The Hidden Feelings of Motherhood, Item 2485 $14.95

The Woman's Book of Sleep, Item 2418 $14.95

Pregnancy Stories, Item 2361 $14.95

The Women's Guide to Total Self-Esteem, Item 2418 $13.95

Thinking Pregnant, Item 2302 $13.95

The Conscious Bride, Item 2132 $12.95

Juicy Tomatoes, Item 2175 $13.95

Call toll free, **1-800-748-6273,** or log on to our online bookstore at www.newharbinger.com to order. Have your Visa or Mastercard number ready. Or send a check for the titles you want to New Harbinger Publications, Inc., 5674 Shattuck Ave., Oakland, CA 94609. Include $4.50 for the first book and 75¢ for each additional book, to cover shipping and handling. (California residents please include appropriate sales tax.) Allow two to five weeks for delivery.

Prices subject to change without notice.